Muay Thai

A Comprehensive Guide to Thai Boxing Basics for Beginners and a Comparison with Dutch Kickboxing

© Copyright 2024 - All rights reserved.

The content contained within this book may not be reproduced, duplicated, or transmitted without direct written permission from the author or the publisher.

Under no circumstances will any blame or legal responsibility be held against the publisher, or author, for any damages, reparation, or monetary loss due to the information contained within this book, either directly or indirectly.

Legal Notice:

This book is copyright protected. It is only for personal use. You cannot amend, distribute, sell, use, quote or paraphrase any part of the content within this book, without the consent of the author or publisher.

Disclaimer Notice:

Please note the information contained within this document is for educational and entertainment purposes only. All effort has been executed to present accurate, up-to-date, reliable, and complete information. No warranties of any kind are declared or implied. Readers acknowledge that the author is not engaging in the rendering of legal, financial, medical, or professional advice. The content within this book has been derived from various sources. Please consult a licensed professional before attempting any techniques outlined in this book.

By reading this document, the reader agrees that under no circumstances is the author responsible for any losses, direct or indirect, that are incurred as a result of the use of the information contained within this document, including, but not limited to, errors, omissions, or inaccuracies.

Table of Contents

INTRODUCTION 1
CHAPTER 1: MUAY THAI RULES AND PHILOSOPHY 3
CHAPTER 2: STARTING WITH STANCE 14
CHAPTER 3: CHOK: PUNCHING TECHNIQUES 24
CHAPTER 4: SOK: ELBOW TECHNIQUES 35
CHAPTER 5: TI KHAO: KNEE TECHNIQUES 45
CHAPTER 6: TE: KICKING TECHNIQUES 56
CHAPTER 7: TEEP: FOOT TECHNIQUES 68
CHAPTER 8: CHAP KHO: CLINCHING AND NECK WRESTLING TECHNIQUES 77
CHAPTER 9: COMBINATION TECHNIQUES 84
CHAPTER 10: DEFENSE TIPS AND TECHNIQUES 91
CHAPTER 11: SPAR LIKE A MASTER 97
CHAPTER 12: MUAY THAI VS. DUTCH KICKBOXING 105
CHAPTER 13: DAILY TRAINING DRILLS 115
CONCLUSION 125
HERE'S ANOTHER BOOK BY CLINT SHARP THAT YOU MIGHT LIKE 127
REFERENCES 128

Introduction

Thailand's rich cultural history has included physical fitness training like Muay Thai for hundreds of years. Many accounts record it as an essential self-defense technique that Thai warriors frequently employed in various battles. The Chupasart wartime manuscript informs using every part of your body is critical to executing effective techniques when battling an opponent with the full commitment of mind, body, and soul.

Kickboxing aims to prepare your body and improve concentration. Therefore, you must train in a somewhat real-life setting. Muay Thai has proved to be the best striking style available in kickboxing. There are other brilliant techniques, like Dutch Kickboxing, but Muay Thai is much more practical and approachable. When you want to build confidence and get physically fit, this is the best sport to be involved in.

Muay Thai is a sport requiring all eight limbs of your body. It focuses on improving concentration and strength in and out of controlled situations. Several techniques are involved, but as a beginner, focusing on building the foundations of your Muay Thai journey is necessary.

This book exposes the philosophy behind Muay Thai and why it is considered the most practical form of Kickboxing, accepted worldwide, especially in the West.

In this book, you learn practical techniques in Thai Kickboxing – Muay Thai, using elbows, knees, arms, legs, kicks, and punches to attack an opponent and using the same means as a defense against them.

This book is a comprehensive yet simple guide taking the reader on a gradual but practical process to applying every technique listed. It's a hands-on approach, and its easy readability sets it apart from others.

This book teaches you that your mind is crucial in building focus and resilience, keeping your stance, and diving more through practice and consistency.

During most training, you would encounter sparing, rhythms, fundamental movements, kicks, jumping knees, and spinning back elbows. You will learn the basics of each and dive into even more advanced styles like uppercuts, head kicks, and spinning elbows. Initially, you might experience very slow development, but with practice and perseverance, improvement will come.

So, grab this opportunity and keep reading to get to the level you desire and master the skill of Muay Thai.

Chapter 1: Muay Thai Rules and Philosophy

Thai boxing, or Muay Thai, is a combat sport with its roots embedded in Thai culture and history. *Muay* translates to "boxing," so Muay Thai translates to Thai boxing. This martial arts form was developed a few hundred years ago, allowing the boxer to use their entire body as a weapon during close combat.

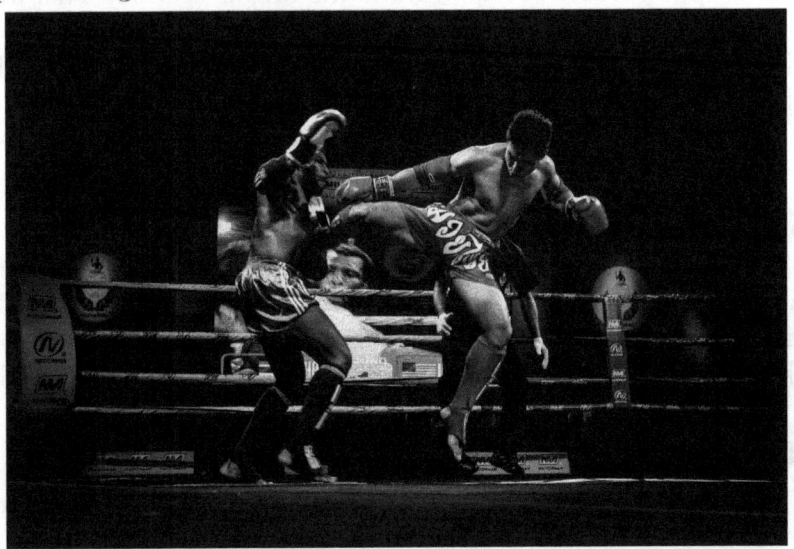

Muay Thai is a close combat sport.
Gerrit Phil Baumann, CC BY 3.0 <https://creativecommons.org/licenses/by/3.0>, via Wikimedia Commons: https://commons.wikimedia.org/wiki/File:Muay_Thai_Fight_Us_Vs_Burma_(80668065).jpeg

Although historians infer that Muay Thai originated centuries ago, no historical record of the sport can be found before the 14th century because of the Burmese invasion and looting. Most of the written history at the time was lost after the Burmese looted Ayudhaya, a capital city in Siam (currently Thailand).

Unlike boxing, throwing knees and hitting the opponent using elbow strikes and kicks is the norm. Furthermore, grappling techniques, initiating throws, and clinching are other techniques allowed and widely practiced in Muay Thai. If you're unfamiliar with Muay Thai, you can easily confuse it with MMA or other forms of combat sports, but there are several differences. The most evident difference giving Muay Thai a unique place in martial arts is the eight points of contact,

Other martial art and combat sports typically have two or four points of contact, whereas Muay Thai follows the art of eight limbs. A fighter can use eight points of contact, allowing punches, knee, and elbow strikes.

This combat sport places a lot of emphasis on cultural aspects, including engaging in the Wai Kru Ram Muay, a pre-fight ritual dance done by Muay Thai fighters, and wearing a Mongkon, a traditional headdress, and playing Sarama music throughout the competition.

This chapter focuses on tapping into the origins of Muay Thai with a brief overview of its history. You read about the philosophy behind this martial arts form and the characteristic features that make Muay Thai stand out from other branches of martial arts.

A Brief History

Before exploring the philosophy behind this powerful fighting style, let's take a quick peek at the history of Muay Thai. The traditional Muay Boran, from which today's Muay Thai was born, was a form of Thai martial arts taught to soldiers to defend the Thai kingdom from enemy attacks and invasions. Due to frequent wars with neighbors, the Muay Thai fighting style became embedded in their culture and lifestyle.

Muay Thai Origins

It originated with the Burmese invasion of Ayudhaya. The invaders plundered what they could put their hands on and turned everything else into ashes. The invading troops took people as prisoners of war. Among these prisoners were a significant number of Thai kickboxers who were held mostly in the city of Ungwa.

Later in the early 1700s, the Burmese ruler honored the Buddha's relics by conducting a seven-day-seven-night celebration. During the celebration days, comedy shows, plays, sword-fighting, and Thai boxing matches were arranged where Thai boxers would compete against Burmese fighters.

The story of Nai Khanom Tom marks the origins of this combat sport. During the celebrations, a Burmese nobleman introduced Nai Khanom Tom to the ring to pit his strength against a Burmese boxer. As a norm, Nai Khanom Tom initiated the pre-fight dance, fascinating the crowd. The Burmese fighter was no match for the veteran Muay Thai boxer as Nai Khanom attacked his opponent fiercely and he collapsed on the ground.

However, the knockout of the Burmese fighter was not considered a victory, and the judges decided that the Thai boxer had to face nine more Burmese fighters as the first one was distracted by the traditional pre-fight dance. Hearing this decision, other Thai boxers held as captives volunteered to fight with Nai Khanom Tom, only to uphold Thai boxing's reputation. His last opponent was a veteran boxing teacher that Nai Khanom Tom used to visit. He, too, was defeated in the fight, after which no other Burmese boxer dared to challenge him.

Upon seeing the courageous and skillful fights, the Burmese ruler wished to reward him. The Muay Thai fighter was given a choice of taking money or beautiful girls as wives, and he chose the Burmese girls. The fighter was released from captivity and sent to his hometown, where he spent the rest of his life.

Now that Muay Thai's history and origin have been covered, let's explore more about modern-day Muay Thai, its principles, and related information to educate you on this robust combat sport.

Modern Muay Thai

The modern form of Muay Thai became the norm in the 20th century, especially after the First World War. The fighting ring and codified rules show how heavily it is influenced by British boxing. Other changes were also accepted, such as wearing gloves instead of wrapping ropes around the hands.

The elements of traditional boxing, like padded boxing gloves, three or five-round limits per game, and the implementation of several rules, shape this combat sport. As mentioned, the fighting style is inspired by the traditional martial arts form of Muay Boran, created for hand-to-hand combat.

Implementing rules that set certain thresholds and limits is necessary since several techniques taught in Muay Boran can be deadly for the opponent when executed. For example, hitting your opponent on the joints or their neck is forbidden. Besides having numerous punch variations like uppercuts and jabs, you can also perform throws, sweeps, and clinching in Muay Thai. Due to the many fighting variations allowed in Muay Thai, it has gained the title of an all-rounded combat sport involving several fighting techniques and protocols from different combat sports.

The Principles of Muay Thai

Whether a veteran in the sport or a newbie, you need a lot of persistence, passion, and dedication to improve. Here are some principles that should be understood and incorporated in your training and life to achieve the best outcomes.

Having a Solid Defense

Instead of working endlessly to perfect your offensive strikes and moves, working on your defense for a well-rounded skill is equally crucial. If you don't have a strong defense, you give the opponent more chances to hit you by allowing openings. Keeping your guard up and anticipating your opponent's next move is key here.

Putting in Effort

Making your best effort and showing dedication is necessary if you expect better results. To be good at the sport, putting in your best when training is crucial.

Working on the Technique

Keep a balance between strength and technique training to achieve your optimum level. You might have seen a Muay Thai fighter knocking out their opponent with a single blow. It seems easy to execute at first, but the fighter puts a lot of dedication and time into perfecting these techniques. To master a technique, start with the basics, like learning the correct stance for the technique, openings during a fight you should look for, and practicing the technique numerous times to build muscle memory and quick reflexes.

Do What You Want

There's no compulsion about how to fight as long as the set rules are followed. Since Muay Thai is a physically challenging sport, training consistently and mastering techniques will only be possible when you enjoy what you're doing. This sheer enjoyment can motivate enough to achieve the set goals on time.

Timing and Distance

Besides working on perfecting techniques and learning new moves, having the correct timing and the right distance is essential in fights. If you don't time your hits well or when the distance is not to the mark, the hit won't make an impact and can result in self-injury.

Following a Plan

When training for Muay Thai, ensure you have a feasible plan. Likewise, in a fight, a Muay Thai fighter can anticipate their opponent's moves after fighting for a few minutes and can instantly develop a viable plan. For example, after the first round, the Muay Thai boxer should initiate a plan, like whether they will distract their opponent with a fake kick or would most likely clinch.

Relaxing the Body

Due to excessive physical activity, the body gets exhausted. In training or a fight, avoiding putting too much strain on the body is necessary. Avoid pushing the body to its limits to avoid injury. Besides training and polishing your skills, rest well and eat nutritious, balanced foods instead of fried and processed foods.

Muay Thai Techniques

Muay Thai uses three basic techniques: attacking, defending, and countering. Consistent practice of these techniques is imperative as it will improve how you use that particular technique and build muscle memory. The training starts with working on the stance and movements to control the body during fights.

The legs are held almost two feet apart, the body is erect, and the hands guard the head. Combatants who favor the right hand will keep their left foot forward and their right foot angled 45 degrees outside. Left-handers will position their right foot ahead and their left foot at an angle.

After the stance and movements are practiced, the next step is to learn attack, defense, and counter moves. The most fundamental attacking moves are clinches, punches, kicks, push kicks, and elbow strikes. Defensive maneuvers include leg catches, dodges, redirecting strikes, leaning back, and blocks. Mixing these basic and other advanced techniques and using them at the right time can win a fighter the game.

Beginners are frequently taught the jab-cross-low kick combination during training. The fighter can progress to practice other advanced techniques and combos. Please remember the techniques shared here are basic and have several variations. Without further ado, let's read about common techniques and their variations.

Punching

It's the most common attack technique in every combat sport, including Muay Thai. Punches have hundreds of variations, but this book only sticks to the established punching techniques and variations. The cross punch (straight rear punch), the jab (straight lead punch), the hook, the spinning back fist, the uppercut, and the overhead punch are some typical punch varieties.

These punching styles have varying stances, as it's the movement that gives power to the punch. For example, a normal punch requires moving the feet quickly by shifting the body weight and rotating the hip and shoulders.

Throwing Kicks

Muay Thai boxers can deliver impactful kicks to devastate their enemy using their shins. Most kicks are initiated from the outside while the opposite arm is swung backward. Simultaneously, the hip joint is rotated to generate force and land an effective kick.

Low kicks are thrown at the opponent's legs, medium kicks at the torso, and high kicks at the head. Besides using the typical roundhouse side kick, Muay Thai has numerous kick variations like spinning back kicks, cartwheel kicks, jumping kicks, and axe kicks, to name a few.

Throwing Elbows

Muay Thai fighters are famous for throwing shin kicks and elbows, as these body parts can deliver an effective blow to the opponent. Several variations are used to throw elbows at opponents, like hitting on the head's side, the chin, from the top down, or in the opposite direction. Other variations include the famous flying elbow and the spinning back elbow that can confuse the opponent to lower their guard and deliver a devastating blow. Perfect elbow strikes have the force to deal serious cuts and swiftly knock the opponent to the ground.

Teep Kicks

In Muay Thai, a push kick is called a *teep kick* and is used for defense and offense. These kicks are mostly used when the opponent is charging in and when you want to create distance for your next offense. The opponent's advances are stopped by using the push kick on the lead leg and torso. Some teeps are aimed at the face and intentionally initiated to show dominance. Teeps can be mixed with kick variations to push the opponent further. Adding a teep to a jumping front kick can push the opponent or cause them to lose their stance.

Knee Throws

Knee throws are the most effective weapon in Muay Thai when in close range or the clinching position. These knee throws mostly aim at the torso, ribcage, thighs, and the opponent's head. Jumping knee strikes are often used in this combat sport and can deliver a knockout blow, ending the fight early.

Clinching

Clinching is a Muay Thai grappling technique combining knee and elbow strikes for maximum damage. While clinching might seem simple at first, it can take several years to master the technique. Clinching can be a game-changing move when executed perfectly, making the opponent tap out in no time.

To improve at Muay Thai, learning these basic techniques and continuously practicing building muscle memory is crucial. Most Muay Thai fighters train twice daily, dividing their practice routine into two parts. The routine is mostly followed year-round except Sundays. As Muay Thai is deeply rooted in Thai culture, it's no surprise to see Muay Thai boxers as young as five years old training to be better at combat sports.

As you start building muscle memory by constantly repeating the techniques, building muscle strength and stamina are equally important. Therefore, cardio and weight exercises are incorporated into a Muay Thai boxer's training routine. This striking balance of strength, agility, and quick reflexes improves a Muay Thai fighter. For beginners, it's best to find a teacher or mentor to build a strong foundation of the philosophy, principles, and practices of Muay Thai.

Benefits of Muay Thai

Although Muay Thai is a combat sport, more people are interested in this sport due to a variety of reasons besides competing in the ring. These reasons include practicing for recreational purposes and improving physical and mental health. Let's review the benefits of practicing Muay Thai for better clarity.

Controlling Calories

As mentioned, combat sport involves cardio, strength exercises, and repeatedly practicing techniques. When executed properly, these training sessions burn calories like no other workout. A typical Muay Thai session lasts at least two hours. It includes a cardio warm-up, a few minutes of shadowboxing, repeating defensive and offensive techniques, and performing numerous strength exercises. These sessions can easily burn more than a thousand calories, making them extremely effective in not only making you lose weight but also developing stamina, endurance, strength, and agility.

Increased Mental Health

Besides improving health, these workouts and training sessions boost mental health. Physical exercise, stamina, and endurance training are some effective methods linked to decreased anxiety, stress, and depression. The exercise, sleep, and diet routine a Muay Thai boxer follows is effective enough to keep stress levels in check and provide clarity when brainstorming.

Improved Self-Defense

Learning attack and defense techniques are the main pillars of Muay Thai. Muay Thai training can help someone inflict damage and defend themselves from harm during close combat because the fighting sport evolved from a previous Thai martial arts style that was created primarily for warfare. Self-defense and disarming tactics include employing offensive techniques, including knee strikes, elbow throws, and push kicks.

Mental Strength

Besides improving mental health, the mental strength of a Muay Thai fighter increases drastically, enabling the boxer to channel their emotions, keep worrisome thoughts at bay, and develop mental fortitude. Muay Thai is about being mentally and physically strong enough to endure adverse and uncertain situations with courage, determination, and a winning attitude.

Endorphin Surge

As Muay Thai involves lengthy training sessions followed by a rest phase to relax and replenish energy, the brain during this relaxation period releases endorphins promoting relaxation and comfort, aiding drastically in managing stress.

Social Bonding

A Muay Thai gym provides a sense of comradeship where you find people striving for the same goals and sharing similar passions. The pain you endure during training with your partners at the gym can forge strong bonds and relationships that can go a long way.

Increased Self-Confidence

With training, your physical appearance improves, boosting self-confidence. A physically strong and appealing body gives you the confidence to not worry about your body shape and be what you truly want to be.

Improved Health

The risk of common medical conditions like cardiovascular diseases, high blood pressure, and diabetes can be reduced through adequate Muay Thai training. Since the sport is cardio-intensive, it improves cardiovascular health and reduces blood pressure.

Besides these benefits, Muay Thai is an amazing combat sport for fitness enthusiasts seeking more than hitting the gym and lifting weights. Instead of repeating the same exercises, you can tweak your routine and learn a new technique or combo.

This last section briefly compares Muay Thai with other popular combat sports forms.

Muay Thai vs. Boxing

Traditional boxing allows punches, but in Muay Thai, you can use knees, elbows, kicks, clinching, and other techniques without restrictions. Both combat sports are ideal for self-defense and competing professionally. Still, it all comes down to personal preference of which combat sport to pursue.

MMA vs. Muay Thai

The most evident difference between these two combat sports is that MMA fighters are more efficient in grappling and use several of these techniques to make their opponent tap out. On the other hand, a Muay Thai boxer will be more efficient in landing impactful strikes.

Brazilian Jiu-Jitsu vs. Muay Thai

Muay Thai is a more athletic combat sport. In contrast, Brazilian Jiu-Jitsu (BJJ) is a more ground fighting and grappling martial art form. Muay Thai fighters believe their techniques can knock out a BJJ fighter instantly. On the other hand, BJJ fighters can use advanced grappling techniques to pin the fighter to the ground and force him to submission.

Key Rules in Muay Thai

There might be slight changes in the rules and regulations, but here are the most common rules virtually every Muay Thai organization follows.

- A standard ring should be between 4.9 by 4.9 meters to 7.3 by 7.3 meters. Adequate cushioning material must be applied on the four corner posts and the floor.
- The official minimum age for a Muay Thai fighter to compete professionally is 15 to 18 years, depending on the country.
- Protective gear like gloves, elbow pads, head guards, and even a padded vest are sometimes mandatory.
- The glove size should be six to ten ounces according to the weight category. Some organizations allow MMA gloves with open fingers between four to six ounces.
- Weigh-ins are carried out one day earlier or on the same day of a fight. Fighters are categorized according to their weight division.
- Only Muay Thai shorts are allowed as apparel for male fighters. Some Muay Thai fighters with strong traditional beliefs wear sacred armbands called *prajiad*.
- Each fight is five three-minute rounds with two-minute breaks after each round. For the casual viewer, some TV programs and sports networks cut the game into three rounds of three minutes each.

- The winner is decided via a scoring system if there is no knockout in a match. The Muay Thai boxer that effectively lands more and inflicts more damage is considered the winner. When a player wins a round, ten points are awarded, and the opponent is given a number lower than ten, depending on their performance in the round.
- A referee has the authority to stop the fight in the case of a knockout or when one Muay Thai boxer clearly overpowers their opponent.
- If the combatant is deemed unfit to continue (which could result in other health problems), the on-call doctor can call off the fight.
- Common offenses that result in a fighter's disqualification include headbutts, groin shots, kicking knee joints, and prodding the eyes.
- Spitting or swearing are also prohibited and can result in a penalty.

Muay Thai has a rich and fascinating history carried through generations and styles to become today's intense and rewarding combat sport.

Chapter 2: Starting with Stance

Muay Thai's foundation lies in the Jot Muay, a crucial element for executing fighting techniques effectively. Without a stable stance, it's impossible to develop advanced combat skills.

Over time, varied fighting postures replaced older ones. Now, many centers train their students using a variant of Western boxing guards regarded as standard everywhere among instructors globally. When looking back at heritage practices, it was discovered that most training camps taught distinct techniques based on geographical location – North, Northeastern, South, or Central Thailand.

But in this chapter, you learn the traditional Muay fighting stances, which is the origin of different techniques and variants used today. This chapter covers detailed instructions for practicing each stance using factors like balance, rhythm, and basic footwork. You learn additional tips for mastering these stances and positions, popular mistakes, and avoiding them.

The Significance of Foot Placement in Muay Thai

If you aim to master Siamese fighting culture, honing your foot's accuracy and precision is a must. According to the age-old customs of Muay Thai martial arts, there are three broad classifications for foot positions: 1-point support, 2-point support, and 3-point support systems, including the triangle stance-imaginary vertices where fighters stand.

Advancing through each position is vital to react promptly against your opponent's movements. The triangle stance is the basis for all other techniques within Muay Thai and underpins its philosophy.

Knowledge about foothold techniques is essential for a comprehensive understanding of this discipline. Therefore, adhering strictly to conventional rules becomes vital in attaining success while perfecting footing practices like standing legs apart at shoulder distance recommended by experts.

Balance is everything in Muay Thai, and proper foot placement makes all the difference. Aim to position your feet so the rear foot is higher than the front to master the art of balance. This stance allows for excellent evasions alongside swift, accurate counterstrikes that pack a punch.

The Significance of Arm Positions

You must master adopting optimal stances that create triangular shapes using the body as a guide to excelling in Muay Thai fighting. This technique enables professionals to move effortlessly while maximizing the potential of their limbs as lethal weapons.

Achieving the desired combat posture necessitates proper hand placement and shielding against vulnerabilities like exposing the throat and opening yourself up to danger from opponents.

In close-quarter encounters, when stability takes precedence over movement or flexibility during long-range encounters, defensive measures must prioritize protecting vulnerable areas like the torso and front regions.

Muay Thai technique execution success is mostly dependent on low gravity center tactics. You must maintain slightly bowed knees, slightly crouching shoulders, slightly spread legs, and an upright chest. These crucial elements provide fighters optimal stability and protect their throats from attacks when engaging opponents head-on.

Traditional Muay Thai Fighting Stances

The five common traditional Muay Thai fighting stances are outlined in this section.

1. Muay Chaiya Fighting Stance

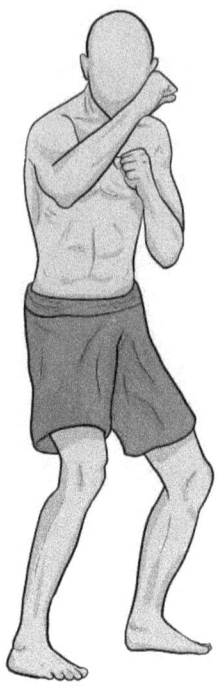

Muay Chaiya stance

Efficiency is key in achieving victory through Muay Chaiya's fighting stance, as advised by Grand Master Khet Sriyaphai. This posture is similar to durian fruits protected by thorns inflicting pain on anything that touches it.

Jot Muay Chaiya can hurt an opponent similarly as long as the stance is done correctly. A fighter must divide their body into six quadrants: left lower, right upper, left upper, right middle, left middle, and right lower. Each requires a unique defensive technique tailored to the corresponding attacks.

Arms defend the upper to middle quadrants, while legs shield the lower ones. Defensive maneuvers aim for maximum efficiency by using the shortest path to cover an endangered quadrant, eliminating wasted motion.

2. Muay Korat

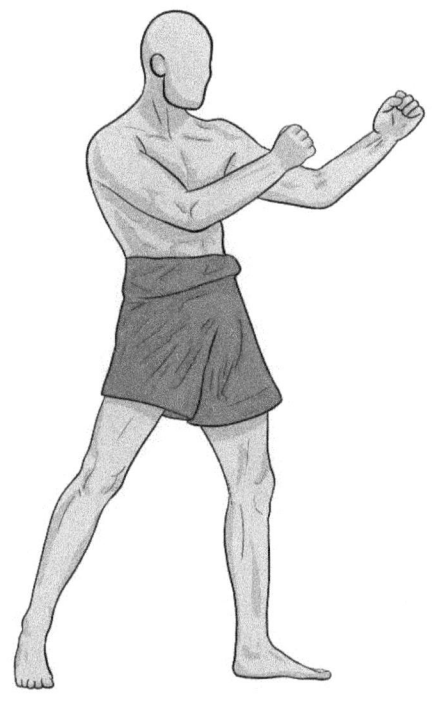

Muay Korat stance.

In contrast to Chaiya, the Muay Korat posture represents an offensive approach. Its structure has been thoughtfully designed to maximize attack effectiveness. Implementing this fighting stance requires assertive and aggressive movements using powerful strikes employing both arms and legs.

Fists should be parallel to your chest with one arm stretched outward to cover a large area in front and block any susceptible openings for an opponent's attack. This position allows for quick, fierce counterattacks. The strong defensive character of this stance allows for quick, lethal counterattacks.

The location of the feet creates an aggressive, commanding posture that places most of the body's weight on the front leg. The rear leg offers stability and support, shortening the space between the knees, which must be kept flexed. The stability of the back leg and the closer knee distance enable quick, aggressive footwork.

3. Muay Lopburi

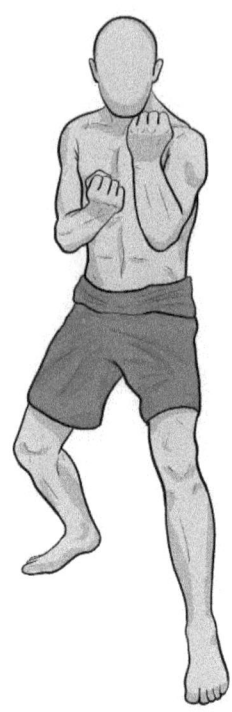

Muay Lopburi fighting stance

The *Muay Lopburi* fighting stance has a unique hand position with fists turned, palms facing upward, and elbows bent. The hands are lower than the other two stances.

Western bare knuckle boxers' guard inspired this stance to enable swift punches, particularly the upward swing punch popular among Lopburi boxers. The positioning of the feet is critical in this stance allowing for flexibility in attack and defense.

You require quick footwork with legs not too far apart to maintain balance and your center of gravity. While defending, the rear foot should be flat but raised while attacking or moving forward to show versatility.

4. Muay Pranakorn

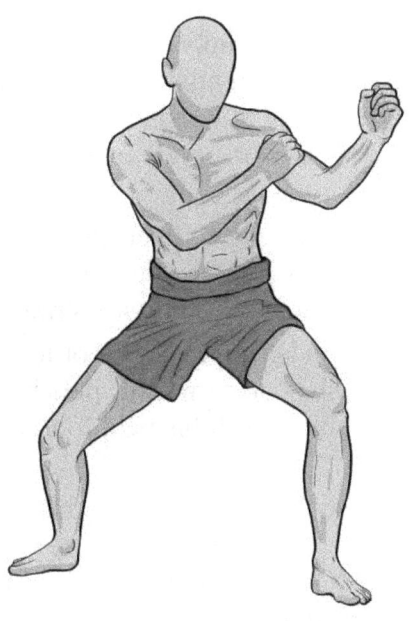

Muay Pranakorn fighting stance

One of the most dynamic postures fighters adopt is known as *Muay Pranakorn*. It borrows specific elements from other styles and combines them to form a well-rounded stance worth mastering.

The most notable aspect of this position is how far apart it keeps each leg, creating ample space between them, standing out immediately upon observation by onlookers or opponents.

While standing firmly, one leg is turned outwards at ninety degrees; the other leg must be centered forward, facing the opponent. The fighter's knees are significantly bent to lower their center of gravity and increase balance.

The benefit of this stance is it makes fighters appear smaller while providing an edge in combat by unsettling their opponents.

Bent at the elbow, the fighter's rear arm offers protection from potential attacks toward the upper body region for added defensive advantage. Its unique formation and defensive capabilities make the Muay Pranakorn stance perfect for launching powerful limb strikes.

Additional Tips for Mastering These Stances

To excel at Muay Thai, you must understand how vital proper positioning is for attacking and defending effectively. If you don't master this skill, sparring sessions might feel more like frustrating exercises than enjoyable ones. Additionally, hitting pads or bags won't produce much force.

Western boxing and Muay Thai combat sports recognize two fighting styles – orthodox or southpaw – depending on whether an athlete uses his left or right hand more often as his primary striking weapon.

The orthodox fighter stands with his left foot forward, relying mostly on his right side to push out powerful punches. Conversely, the southpaw fighter typically stands with his right foot forward, using his left arm for the attack.

Interestingly, some Muay Thai fighters showcase their preferred side by wearing ankle straps. Some choose one strap on the stronger foot, while others might choose an eye-catching anklet contrasting with their shorts' hue at the opposite ankle.

But whether they're southpaws or orthodox athletes, correct body positioning remains crucial if you want maximum power output and success rates.

Here are several essential factors in establishing an unwavering foundation anyone should consider as they enhance their personal approach to achieving top-notch results in Muay Thai.

Elbow, Head, and Hands Positioning

The wrong elbow, head, and hands positions may get you seriously hurt – no matter how cool you might think you look!

To properly position yourself and make your hands hang down naturally, bring both thumbs level with your eyebrows and your palms facing each other.

Achieving optimal results requires careful attention to form, including positioning your elbows slightly farther apart than your hands. But don't force anything; you don't want to feel like you're pushing or pulling any part of your body into an uncomfortable or unnatural position.

Your hands should be touching your forehead, and you should tuck in your chin just enough to safeguard it with both shoulders in case a punch comes flying at you from either side. Don't tilt too much but keep your chin up.

With your stance and bodily alignment in check, it's time to focus on refining footwork techniques for optimal performance.

Footwork

Maintaining proper form is key for a good stance in martial arts training. While it's typically recommended fighters keep their feet slightly apart, at least shoulder width or wider, exceptions like those of fighter Nong O Gaiyanghadao, who varies foot distance throughout fights, cannot be overlooked.

By taking a wider stance during some fights as part of deflections and strikes, he maintains balance under pressure, absorbing incoming kicks better than with the narrower foot placement used during Teep strikes.

For those beginning martial arts, start with a good foundational stance that has your feet more than shoulder width apart while staying steady on your feet with knees bent and flexed. As you become more comfortable in your foundation, experiment with different foot distances to determine what works best while maintaining a solid center of balance.

You should keep your hips directly facing the opponent's and not sideways like a boxer. Always adjust your foot position based on the technique you plan to use for optimal results while keeping good form at all times.

A crucial point to remember is this principle is also true for your hands and arms. Work harmoniously with your footwork and overall game plan to attain peak performance.

Mistakes to Avoid During Stance

The Fighting Stance is a topic ripe for debate within Muay Thai circles concerning what constitutes the best posture and approach in combat. However, critical errors can significantly impair your performance. This section looks closely at some mistakes.

1. Poor Flexibility and Adaptability

Flexibility and adaptability are essential to succeed with a proper fighting stance because there isn't a single universal stance that applies across all situations. It's about adapting to specific circumstances rather than relying on a particular approach or style. Always be ready to strike while protecting vulnerable areas of the body from an opponent's attack.

Depending on the situation, you might stand up straighter for techniques like sidekicks or assume a lower profile with heightened protection for better defense against incoming blows.

What happens when special opportunities present themselves tactically? Sometimes intentionally lowering your guard could lure an unwary opponent right into your counterattack trap.

The bottom line is to stay aware of the context and adapt accordingly with flexibility to changing circumstances. Flexibility is key to being successful in combat. Avoid getting anchored down by a rigid fighting stance. Be ready and willing to modify your tactics based on the scenario.

2. Neglecting the Neck

Neglecting the protection of the neck area when adopting a fighting stance is a prevalent mistake among many martial artists or combat sports practitioners. Getting punched in this vulnerable region can have severe consequences like concussions or death.

Consciously be aware that it must not be overlooked or neglected at any cost. Hence prioritizing its defense becomes imperative while devising or adopting a sub-discipline-related approach like Thai boxing or kickboxing techniques.

A proper fighting stance entails raising the arms while tucking in the chin securely and leaning forward to provide optimal protection for the neck region. However, novices often overlook this aspect while keeping their hands up, which can have detrimental effects.

Therefore, during sparring sessions or training drills, focus primarily on shielding your neck effectively. Once this objective is achieved, other necessary aspects of a complete fighting stance will follow naturally.

3. Not Relaxing

When attempting Thai boxing or kickboxing for the first time, many people struggle to balance tension and relaxation on the mat. It is understandable; making quick moves while staying cool under pressure takes time and practice. So, what's the solution?

One trick is to imagine yourself feeling completely spent after running an arduous marathon. Let yourself sink into complete exhaustion before gradually raising your arms toward your chin, remaining as loose as possible throughout every motion. It might be tough at first, but mastering this level of relaxation is essential for improving your Thai boxing performance.

Whether an experienced fighter or just starting in the world of Thai boxing, perfecting your fighting stance is critical for success. A strong stance enables more efficient executions of attack and defense movements. But it's not only about holding a fixed position.

In reality, fighting stances are adopted during transitional moments between movements requiring flexibility and fluidity to execute properly. Different combat sports have unique rules regarding which strikes are permitted within competition settings. Therefore, diverse stances have been developed to fit specific needs.

By honing your understanding of these techniques and exploring those that work best for your particular style, you'll boost your chances of coming out on top in a contest.

Chapter 3: Chok: Punching Techniques

Even though Muay Thai is known worldwide as the "Art of Eight Limbs," punches are an important aspect of the sport. Punches for this sport were once limited, relying mostly on knees, kicks, clinching, and basic punching techniques.

However, things have changed, and boxing is now fundamental in the sport, putting fighters restricted to their hands at a disadvantage. Numerous Muay Thai stars are recognized for their techniques, expertise, and sudden and rapid punches. Saensak Muangsurin, Veeraphol Sahaprom, and the famous Samart Payakaroon are examples of fighters who succeeded when progressing from Muay Thai to boxing.

The Major Punching Techniques

Muay Thai has been imbued with Western boxing styles, and the development of punching techniques resulted from this combination. Currently, these punching techniques are broken down into 8 major types. The descriptions of the punches below are explained from the view of a typical fighter. If you fight orthodoxly, the punches would be performed with the opposing feet, hands, and limbs.

1. The Jab

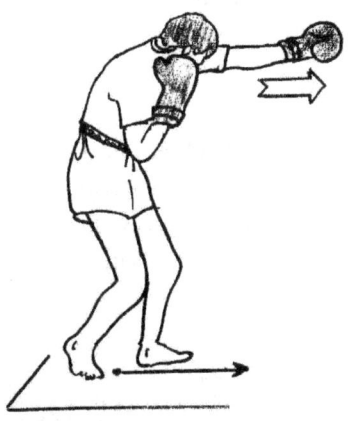

The jab is the easiest punch.
Alain Delmas (France), CC BY-SA 3.0 <http://creativecommons.org/licenses/by-sa/3.0/>, via Wikimedia Commons: https://commons.wikimedia.org/wiki/File:Jab3.jpg

The jab is widely used in Muay Thai and boxing, making it the most significant in the sport. It is the easiest punch and very important, unlike in boxing, where it does not assure dominance. As a beginner in Muay Thai, your trainer will certainly dwell on improving the jab. It works for defense and offense. Various combinations can be set up from the jab, helping a fighter maintain distance from the opponent.

Why is jab frequently used? It is the fastest punch to deliver and is usually the punch to throw when within reach of your opponent. A jab is handy for countering an opponent who keeps advancing toward you aggressively. You require strength to throw an excellent jab. When used correctly, it can be a technique to throw your opponent's combination into disarray. Also, jabs can initiate other moves and punches. Your opponent is within reach and open to further attacks once your jab hits.

To counter the jab, you must paw or parry it with the aid of the high hand on the right. Then, you can push your jab up front, with just a little jab step, as it is parried off. Boxers use an effortless act of ducking to safeguard themselves from jabs. Ducking is a movement to get around and disorient your opponent.

How to Throw a Jab

When throwing a jab, launch your shoulders forward when punching to produce a nice snap so that your jaw and shoulder meet. It increases the jab's reach, and your shoulders shield your chin. As you extend your fists, let your knuckles face upwards and your palm downward while your elbow stretches. Don't forget to bend your knees a little during the punch and pop back up after you've delivered your jab. Your balance would be off if your knees were straightened, lessening the power and control in your jab.

Always keep your rear hand close and tight to your face when throwing the jab with your lead hand. If you drop your guard, you are left wide open for the opponent to throw a left hook. Also, remember your stance must be correct to throw a good jab.

2. The Cross

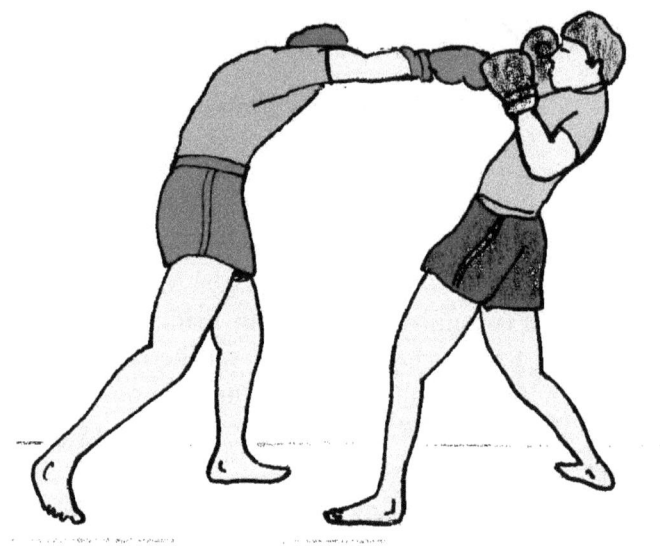

The cross travels farther than a jab.
Delmas Alain, CC BY-SA 3.0 <https://creativecommons.org/licenses/by-sa/3.0>, via Wikimedia Commons: https://commons.wikimedia.org/wiki/File:Retrait4color.jpg

The cross, known as the straight punch, is a powerful punch launched from the backhand. It is usually used as a punch to knock out the opponent in Muay Thai. Although used regularly, like the jab, it is not regularly used as a punch to set up combinations. It is thrown mostly after a combination or a jab. Unlike the jab, the cross does not immediately connect after throwing it. Also, it travels the farthest.

The cross punch is made with the hand furthest from the opponent. This distance and the potential to add rotational force and weight to the strike make it one of your strongest punches. The cross can ward off your opponents because it is a very strong punch. When a good cross connects with an opponent's chin, it can knock them out or at least stun them.

Jabs can be countered with a cross. The cross is excellent for landing power punches on an opponent's outside and can be launched before or after a low kick. You can combine or add it to normal punch and kick combinations. The trick to throwing a great cross is to begin with a body punch to lower your opponent's guard and create the opening to land your shot.

How to Throw a Cross

The common setup for a cross is to give a hard, fast jab first. The trick is to drive your right toe into the ground while rotating your body as you bend your knees and lean your upper body forward slightly to align with your opponent. Then, throw the punch with your thumbs rotated downward, facing the floor, and following your elbow as it extends. Also, ensure your rear foot is pivoted while throwing a cross; when you do this correctly, your heel will be upwards with your toes on the ground, facing the exact direction your punch is headed. You must do everything in one motion so your body's power goes with the punch. Then, quickly return the hand to avoid a counter.

3. The Hook

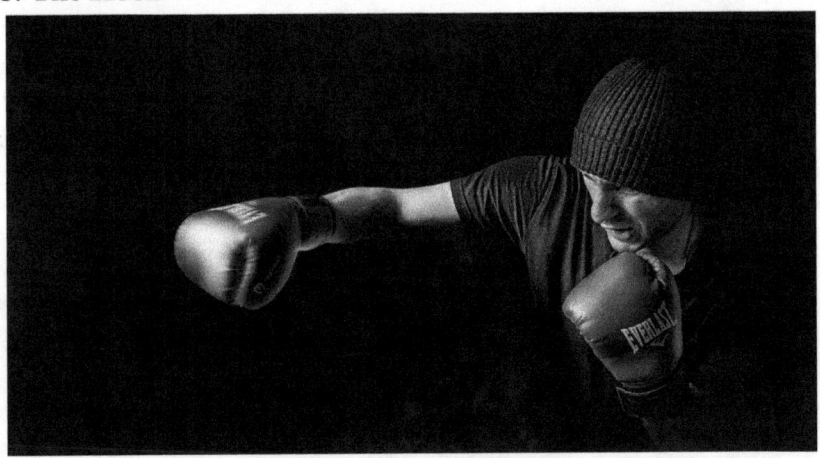

A hook is a difficult punch to perfect.
https://www.pexels.com/photo/man-doing-boxing-163403/

Your opponent's sides can be attacked with the hook. It is delivered with your leading or rear hand. Launching a hook with your leading hand is a great strategy to catch an opponent with good movement, and it is difficult to see if you can lure the opponent into a trap. By the time you have mastered the technique, it can be launched easily and even delivered while jumping.

It is widely known and used in Muay Thai, even though it is the most difficult punch to perfect. A bad-hooking technique can lead to a fractured wrist and even back pain. The hook delivered with the rear hand can often knock out your opponent and is very hard to disguise. It is commonly thrown in close range to your opponent. Still, it leaves you open to counterattacks if the timing is off and launched carelessly. However, it is a good way to end a fight. Before backing up, launch a hook at your opponent's head and finish with a shot to his ribs.

The left hook is regularly used in combinations. Like the cross, a hook is not a long-range shot to reach your opponents. Therefore, it is infrequent for a right-footed fighter to launch a right hook in their basic stance. Suppose you throw a right hook in a right-foot stance; your fist would be inches from your lead hand. It doesn't make right hooks impossible; they are just not as conventional as the left hook.

How to Throw a Hook

Adjust your body weight to your back leg from a correct stance while bending your knees slightly. At the same moment, turn your body with your hips, transferring all the kinetic energy to the punch. Bend your arm at an angle of 90 degrees while placing your elbow just behind your lead hand to land the punch with the elbow of your lead hand bent and your knuckles and closed fist pointing to the ground. The shoulder, elbow, and hand must all be in a line. To boost the punch's force, rotate with your lead foot simultaneously while your right-hand guards your chin for defense.

4. The Uppercut

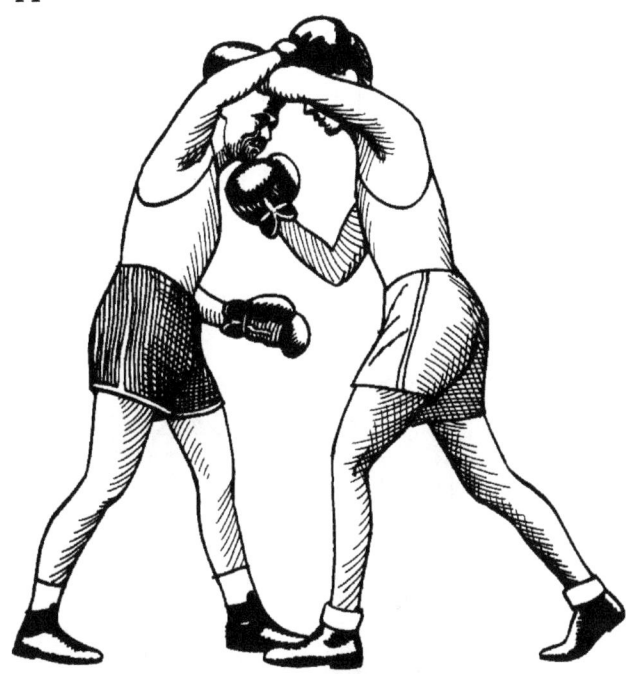

An uppercut is an attack aimed at the chin.
https://commons.wikimedia.org/wiki/File:Uppercut_(PSF).png

Those who disagree that the hook is the most powerful blow in Muay Thai usually claim it is the uppercut. The execution method of this punch is similar to the hook, but the angle of attack is aimed at the chin. A tricky punch, the uppercut can incur great damage if it connects. Imagine having a hard smack on your chin; it can throw you off balance and achieve a knockout if the force is powerful enough.

The uppercut can be brutal and devastating during close combat, but connecting your opponent with it from the outside is difficult. It is rarely used as starting or lead punches because it can be detected, blocked, or countered easily. Due to the skill and timing needed to master this shot, it is the hardest blow to land.

If you practice Muay Thai, you should perfect your hook and know that landing this punch leaves you open to elbows and front kicks.

To deliver an uppercut, you must ensure producing an upward motion does not disrupt your defense. First, turn before adjusting your weight to the side where you hit from, before bringing up your looped arm toward the opponent's jaw or chin.

How to Counter an Uppercut

The two common mistakes that open you to uppercuts are not taking the right stance, exposing your chin, and overextending your blows. Being in the proper stance and having your techniques closed helps guard against your opponent's uppercuts. To counter an uppercut, you must launch a jab when your opponent punches. Many fighters move forward before delivering the uppercut, so you must catch them immediately. The step is taken as soon as their head crosses the centerline.

5. The Swing

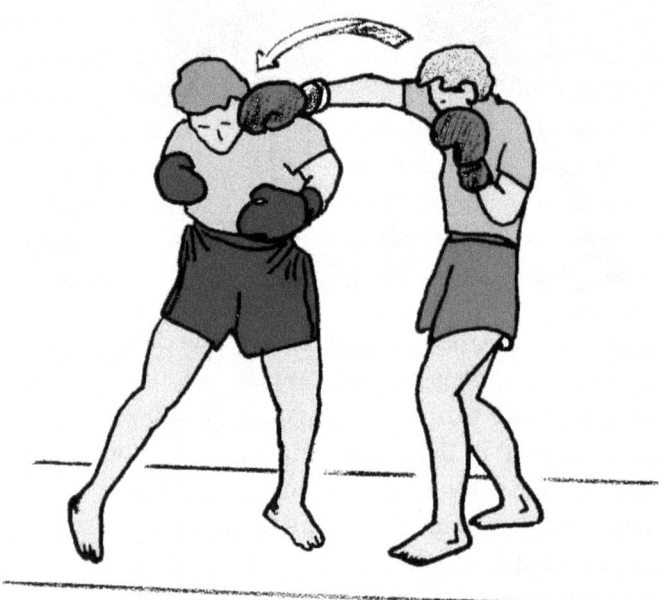

The swing's movement is similar to the hook.
Delmas Alain, CC BY-SA 3.0 <https://creativecommons.org/licenses/by-sa/3.0>, via Wikimedia Commons: https://commons.wikimedia.org/wiki/File:Drop4color.jpg

The swing's movement is almost the same as the hook, but the arm is more extended. The punch is best understood as being more of a swipe. Its capability of reach makes up for its inadequacy in power. A fighter can reach far when they throw the swing delivering an attack to the opponent's side. Like the hook, it is not often launched with the backhand or used as a lead punch. A jab or another strike usually conceals this swing. Also, it is not used in close combat because it is far-reaching.

The swing is not regarded as a punch for a knockout because it lacks power, but it is a good technique to catch your opponent off guard. It's uncommon to deliver a hooked blow from a distance. However, catching opponents when they're off guard is a good attack and makes them nervous. The swing is useful for fighters lacking in height because it helps them close the distance.

You must keep your distance to counter a fighter who swings wildly; if you cannot, try blocking, but not for long. A barehanded blow can easily pass a block. So, quickly step back and rush toward the legs below the knee to take the opponent down.

6. Overhand Punch

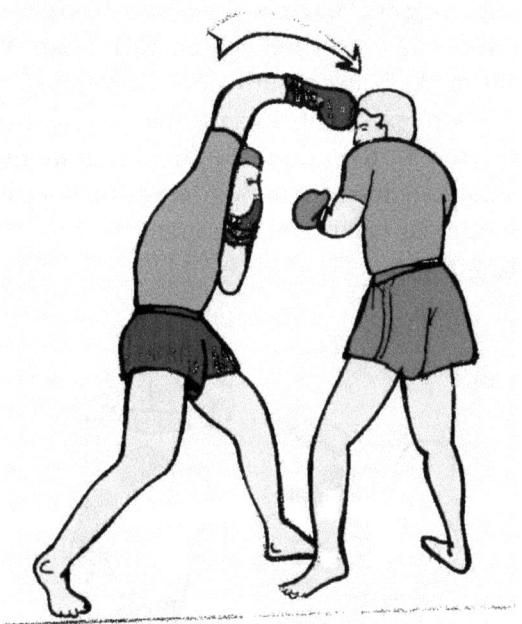

The overhand punch is tricky to learn.
Alain Delmas France), CC BY-SA 3.0 <https://creativecommons.org/licenses/by-sa/3.0>, via Wikimedia Commons: https://commons.wikimedia.org/wiki/File:Drop1color.jpg

The overhand punch is another hook punch, launched from behind and looping over the head. It can knock the opponent out if executed properly with sufficient power. However, this technique is very tricky to learn.

The two disadvantages to this technique are:
- If you fail to hit, your balance will be off, and you will be wide open for counterattacks.

- The blow is not easy to deliver when you are up against left-handed fighters because their head, which is your target, is far away.

This technique works well when fighting taller opponents because it can surprise them and override their defenses. A good combination where to use this punch is after a left-leg onside kick. A suitable way to counter this technique is to tilt backward, launching your punch before your opponent returns to their stance. Raising your left hand upward, like picking up a phone, can block the overhand punch.

How to Throw an Overhand Punch

Suppose the distance between you and your opponent is shrinking, and you see an opening to land an overhand. In that case, it must be done quickly and directed at your opponent's head. You must bend your elbows at an angle between 90-135o, depending on the distance between you and your opponent. Ensure the punch comes above your shoulder and head in a loop motion to guide the strike downward as you lean slightly outside your lead foot. Bending your knees simultaneously as you strike to keep your balance is important.

7. Spinning Back Fist

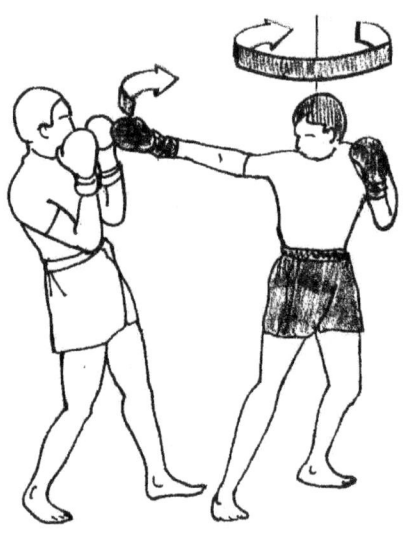

The spinning back fist is an advanced technique.
Delmas Alain, CC BY-SA 3.0 <https://creativecommons.org/licenses/by-sa/3.0>, via Wikimedia Commons: https://commons.wikimedia.org/wiki/File:Spin-back-fist.jpg

This technique is advanced. The motion and movements are unique to other punches mentioned. To counter this technique, duck as your opponent throws it or keep a high guard, rotate your head, and launch a counter hook.

How to Throw a Spinning Back Fist

To throw a spinning back fist, do the following:

- Take a step turning your body. Those who fight conventionally would take a step to the right with their lead.
- Then, raise your right leg, turning around with your left while your right arm is fully extended.
- Hit your opponent using the backside of your hand or the base of your fist.
- The rotating action with the centrifugal force from the spin gives this punch a powerful impact. If this technique is executed properly, it will carry a lot of power and knock out your opponent if it connects.

8. Superman Punch

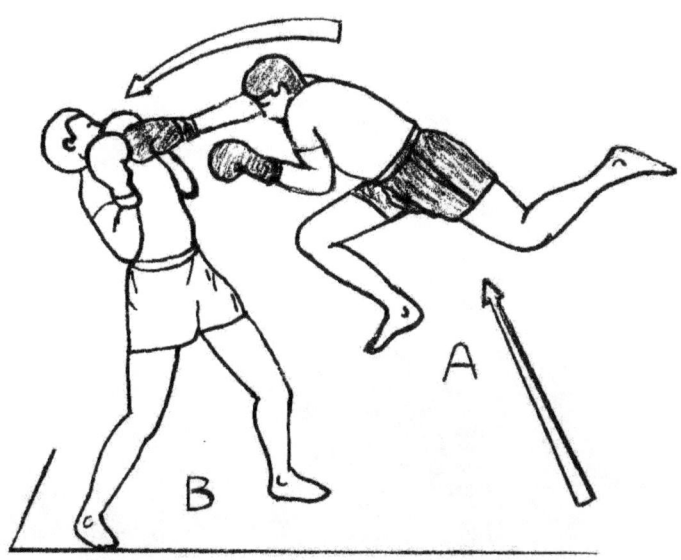

The superman punch is also known as the flying punch.
Delmas Alain, CC BY-SA 3.0 <https://creativecommons.org/licenses/by-sa/3.0>, via Wikimedia Commons: https://commons.wikimedia.org/wiki/File:Flying-punch.jpg

This technique is a basic flying overhand punch. Even though people feel it's a spectacular technique, it is not the strongest punch. It can be easily countered because it is quickly detected once launched.

To counter a Superman punch, deflect it or step out of the way.

How to Throw a Superman Punch

To throw a Superman punch:
- You must fake a kick before leaping into the air
- Launch your hand forward in the air, stretching your leg out simultaneously

This technique is suitable against tall opponents because it reduces the distance and gets past their defense. The punch should not be frequently executed because it is very exposed, making it easy to counter.

Practice makes everything perfect; this old saying is never incorrect. Ensure you use these techniques regularly. The Superman and spinning punches might seem cool but do not affect opponents if executed incorrectly. When used by an inexperienced fighter, the counterattacks will be executed easily. Try not to execute these techniques until you are confident in your ability to do them correctly, thus *effectively*.

Chapter 4: Sok: Elbow Techniques

The Muay Sok in Thailand means "elbow fighter." The fighter focuses on being in close range with his opponent in Muay Sok. The aim is to avoid many kicks and catch the opponent off balance to deliver a nice sharp elbow strike. Whoever closes the distance has a better chance to ring off the target and force them to fight in the suitor's range.

What makes this technique so unique is the level of aggression. The Muay Sok fighter uses different elbow strikes to succeed in various positions. There are several elbow strikes, including *sok ping* (spare elbow), *sok tad* (horizontal elbow), *sok ngad* (uppercut elbow), *sok ti* (slashing elbow), and *sok klap* (spinning elbow). These strikes are used differently, i.e., horizontal, diagonal upward and downward, uppercuts, etc.

This chapter exposes you to the different practical ways to apply each technique, creating a defense system from an opponent's attack and making a counterattack. You learn the minor mistakes you will likely encounter as a beginner and how to overcome them.

What separates this kickboxing technique from others is the elbow strikes. These strikes can knock out an opponent at a shorter range and deliver a bladed cut or blow to the target's face. This is the uniqueness of Must Sok, which no other fighting style employs.

How to Use the Elbow Strikes

The elbow is so sharp and hard that it can give a blunt cut to your target's skin if you attack at a close range or ground level. The elbow strike works effectively as a counterattack for an opponent's punch. Due to these multiple benefits, the elbow strike should be implemented as a style for every self-defense mechanism.

In martial arts, just throwing your elbows to hit an opponent's face is not as effective as applying a few other brutal techniques. In Muay Thai boxing, the elbows are used in various ways: horizontal motion, vertical upward motion, vertical downward motion, an uppercut, backward spinning movement, and the flying elbow. The elbow can attack your target's face from the side, and this could cut their brow. The vertical elbows are more efficient in speed, although not as fast as the others.

The elbow strikes are executed in two ways; the single elbow and the follow-up elbow. However, there's a great distinction between both. The single elbow is independent of other strikes, while the follow-up is done with the same arm on the same target. For example, throwing a punch and immediately striking your opponent with an elbow. However, elbows are only used when the distance between opponents is small. Elbows are a good defense against side knees, body kicks, punches, etc.

In Muay Thai boxing, there are nine elbow strikes, including;

- **Sok Tad (Horizontal Elbow)**

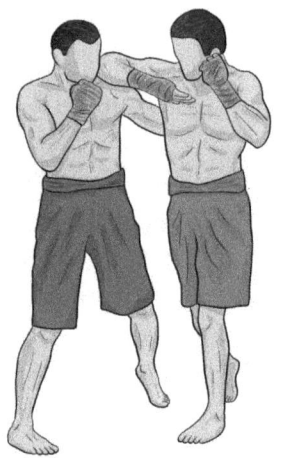

Sok Tad is similar to a hook.

The horizontal elbow is the easiest and most popular elbow strike. This elbow strike can be likened to a hook punch. How is that possible? When you strike, turn your hips, and move the feet on the lead side of your body to deliver the blow. Keep your other arm over your face during this strike to protect against counterattacks. The aim of this movement is directed toward the target's chin and lower face. You can use this move to breach the defense of your opponent.

- **Sok Ngad (Uppercut Elbow)**

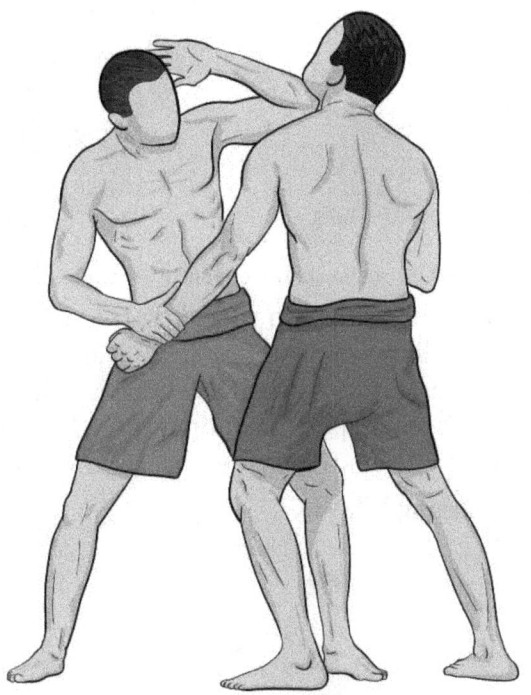

Sok Ngad is one of the fastest strikes in Muay Thai.

The uppercut elbow is one of the most striking and fastest elbow strikes in Muay Thai. This strike is quick and lands a sharp blade cut on the target. Using this can weaken your opponent's defense. How is this possible? With the uppercut elbow, you strike your elbow between your opponent's arms aiming directly for their chin. It can result in a clean knockout blow.

- **Sok Ti (Slashing Elbow)**

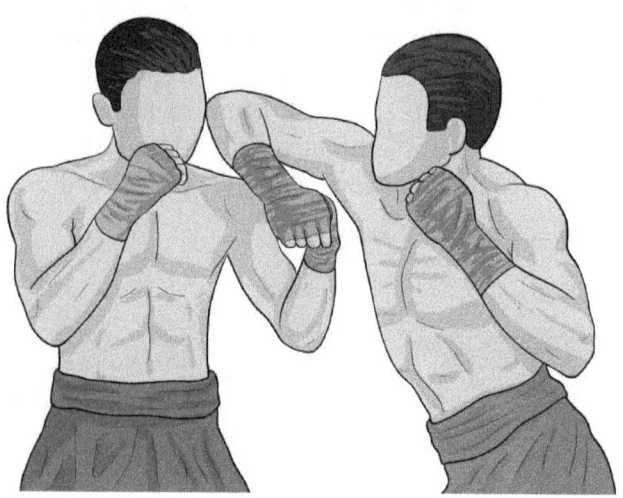

Sok Ti can break your opponent's defense.

This elbow movement is thrown in a slicing downward motion. The target point for this strike is the forehead, the cheeks, or directly above your opponent's eyes. This strike is effective in breaking your opponent's defense. Your opponent will put up a defense to block your attack, but you can wear them out if you keep striking with your elbow.

- **Sok Klap (Spinning Elbow)**

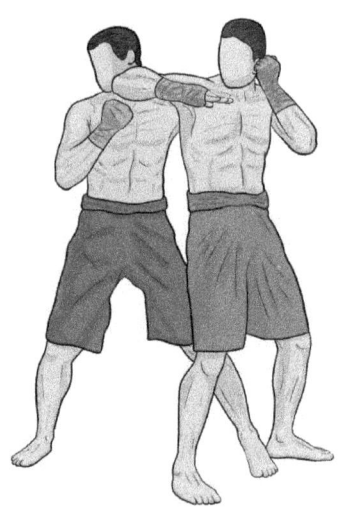

Sok Klap is a classic Muay Thai move.

This movement is a classic move in Muay Thai. It takes a level of mastery of the previous techniques to apply this one. This technique requires care as it must be performed with your back turned against your opponent while striking with the other elbow. Do not underestimate this move, as it can effectively land a knockout blow to the target. How do you apply it? Step your feet across your opponent's side and rotate your upper torso. Use the rear elbow to land a blow to the side of the target's face. Ensure to observe your target from the side of your shoulder while executing this strike, and rotate back immediately after you land the strike.

- **Sok Phung (Forward Elbow Thrust)**

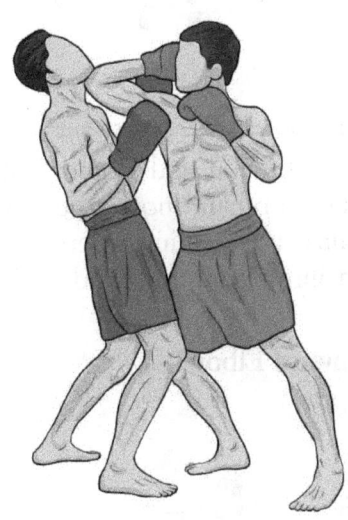

Sok Phung is similar to the uppercut elbow.

This elbow movement is often mistaken for the uppercut elbow. The only distinction between both is that the elbow is thrown forward instead of upward in the forward thrust, as in an uppercut. How do you apply it? Step toward your opponent, pushing them with your hip. Set up your elbow like a spear and thrust it into the target.

- Sok Ku (Double Elbow)

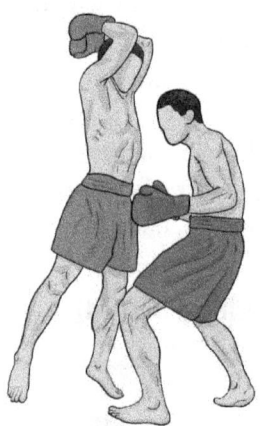

Sok Ku can help you eliminate your opponent

This is a fantastic movement, and when used properly can make a smart move. It could be a brilliant move to end your opponent. During combat, once you realize an opening where your opponent might be weak or hurt, you can jump high and land both elbows on the top of their head.

- Sok Tong (Downward Elbow)

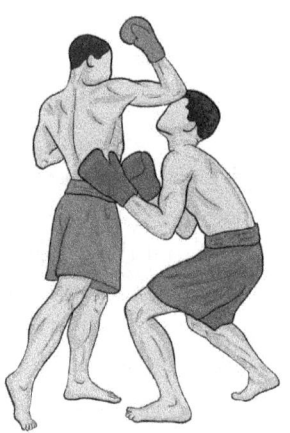

Sok Tong is not commonly used in combat.

This strike is often known as the "12-6" strike because the landing of the elbow resembles the clock reading 12-6. This elbow strike isn't commonly used during combat and is banned in some matches. It is applied similarly to Sok Ku. In this technique, you hit your opponent's thigh, catch his kick, and strike it with your elbow.

Blocking Elbow Strikes

Muay Thai is kickboxing using several clinching techniques, including blocking. Blocking is a crucial defense mechanism skill requiring you to protect your opponent's strikes with your arms, legs, or dodging. In defense, your arms and hands absorb the defects from your opponent's strike. There are other defensive methods in blocking, such as weaving or slipping.

An elbow strike is one of the most powerful strikes in Muay Thai. These strikes usually aim at the target's face, neck, or body. With this strike, you can cut your opponent, causing them to bleed and get distracted. It requires a precise and careful application to be effective. You use your elbow to block another fighter's kick or punch. You bring down your elbow to shield a side of your body using a good fighting stance. To master the art of self-defense, you must first learn to block punches with the shoulder, arm, or elbow so the force's effect is lessened on those sensitive areas of your body.

Due to the hardness of the elbow, it'll take an experienced fighter to use it effectively to knock out or cause harm to their targets since it is difficult to hit with an elbow. They are more effective in a combined attack with punches or kicks, allowing close-range attacks. Learning to block elbow attacks with your forearms and shoulders is essential. Blocking places you in a good position to counterattack with the same arm as soon as your opponent's elbow touches you.

Common Elbow Mistakes Made and How to Overcome Them

Muay Thai is an art new to the Western world. Elbow strikes aren't practiced often because the elbow strike is a very sharp and dangerous technique that can cause injuries and harm easily. The elbow strike is only allowed when competing under the full Thai or MMA rules. However, this does not mean the elbow strike technique should be discarded but used under careful practice without error. Beginners must know the "do's and don'ts" before venturing into this technique. Below are a few elbow strike mistakes beginners and advanced fighters make and how to strengthen them.

Flaw 1: Over Swinging of the Arm

A common mistake is swinging your arm excessively to hit your opponent. This technique adds little or no advantage to a fighter, giving the strike from the elbow more strain and less impact. The goal is to get close to your target and make your upper body flexible enough to turn and land an elbow strike precisely and directly on the target. So, instead of swinging your arm excessively, allow your upper body to be flexible in turns.

It can be difficult resisting using an elbow, but ensure your upper body can turn and engage, so your elbow can connect with the target.

Flaw 2: Leaving the Chin Unprotected

This is a common mistake when punching. While focusing on reading and targeting your opponent, you might lose focus on yourself and leave your chin unguarded; this takes a great toll when there's a counterattack. When reading your opponent and attacking with a punch, ensure your upper arm is folded over your chin in a scarf-like manner. When your opponent counterattacks, your arm shields your face from getting hit.

It is especially important because elbow strikes are in very close range, making it easy for you to get caught off guard when using one.

Flaw 3: Flaring Up the Elbow

Beginners are majorly affected by this. Elevating your elbow before hitting a target when throwing an elbow makes them aware of your stance before you make it. Your elbow should be up with your stance toward the target before you turn and make contact with the target. This move makes it difficult for your opponent to predict your next move.

Flaw 4: A Hard Blow

You might want to land a hard strike to finish your opponent, but using the elbow would cause greater damage, reducing the effects on your hands. Your hands are fragile and can easily get broken, but an elbow is a strong piece of bone, and with it, you can cause significant harm to the target. The best way to use an elbow is horizontal or vertical whipping.

Flaw 5: Fist Clenching

This mistake is common at all levels, beginner and advanced. You don't throw an elbow with your fist clenched; this is poor performance and creates tension on the forearm muscle, making a fighter produce an awkward elbow swing. How to solve it? Keep your hands and fingers loose or relaxed when throwing an elbow. It creates a fluid movement of the arm and allows free motion of the hands.

Tips and Techniques in Sok

First, you must be familiar with the basic techniques. With consistent practice, these techniques grow to cause real harm to your opponent when applied carefully. Basic techniques include the hook, uppercut, spiking elbow, horizontal elbow, and spinning back elbow.

Elbows can be applied in a close or clinch position regardless of the distance. The most essential aspect is that your strike is strong enough to affect your opponents. Here are tips on how to better use the elbow technique:

- Move your hips explosively toward the opponent: While learning punches and kicks, you should also learn to drive your hips explosively toward the opponent to deliver a close-range elbow shot. In an attempt to strike, dig down from your hip to generate more energy for an elbow strike. Your elbow becomes stronger when you learn to move your hips explosively.
- Stabilize your lower back: The muscles on your lower back, when strengthened, stabilizes your hip rotation, allowing efficient movement of the shoulders. To create power, imagine freely thrusting your shoulders at an opponent with a strong elbow strike.
- Keep your shoulders relaxed and flexible: To transfer the energy your hips generate into your elbow, you must learn to relax your shoulders. The body has worked hard to create the energy, so your shoulders must align to strengthen your elbows.

Muay Sok is a crucial aspect of Thailand kickboxing and uses the elbow to strike an opponent. This aspect of combat is what separates it from all other kickboxing forms. The elbow, one of the hardest parts of the body, is used as a weapon and can only be fired at short range and in clinching. It can be dangerous when used correctly and precisely.

This technique can be applied and countered in various ways. As a beginner in Muay Thai, you must learn the basic techniques, master each level, and then progress to other areas of the game. Relying only on an instructional manual would not have as much effect as hitting the gym and registering under a coach. Most importantly, practice is key to mastery.

Chapter 5: Ti Khao: Knee Techniques

Under ancient Thai rule, the knee technique was a highly regarded, high-scoring move. When properly executed, it can leave your opponents with their faces on the ground. In Muay Thai, the knee gives the most prominent and all-round strike capable of giving you victory in a fight. The anatomical part of the knee responsible for perfectly executing this move is your kneecap (patella). It usually works best and produces the most devastating effect.

You observe your kneecap moving as you sit down with your leg straightened on the floor or while standing straight. But when you bend it against the femur, or as if you're striking a Kungfu pose with your leg lifted at an angle, you will notice the kneecap becomes firm. Ensure your heel is up to your butt when attacking while the other leg's toes point to the ground, then hit with your kneecap. This positioning makes it easy to attack your opponent, and driving this striking point with precision and the force coming from your hip makes the strike more effective.

Muay Thai Knee Techniques

Muay Thai, without a doubt, has the best knee techniques in all martial arts. Below are some with the potential to render an opponent unconscious, break their ribs, trigger paralysis, or leave them seriously injured:

The Straight Knee Technique (Khao Trong)

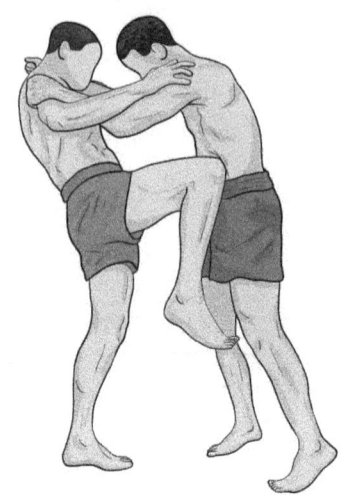

Khao Trong is the simplest knee technique in Muay Thai.

As a beginner, this is the simplest and the most direct knee technique in Muay Thai. The straight knee can be delivered from within or outside the double collar tie (the clinch) and is mostly aimed at your opponent's midsection, striking below the sternum. While it might seem easy, do not let the simplicity of this striking technique throw you off because, when executed correctly, it causes excruciating pain to your opponent's midsection.

If you can use the upward thrust and momentum when you lock your hands behind your opponent's skull, the strike's impact will be more severe. Every goal-oriented fighter must learn the trick behind this technique.

Here are a few tips when using this technique;
- Move forward while stretching forth a leg.
- Thrust your hips forward to generate force by acquiring momentum.
- Target your opponent's upper abdomen while extending your knee diagonally; this improves your strike's effectiveness.
- You must lean back to increase your force.
- Protect your chin by tucking it into your chest.

- When landing from your hit, your kneeling shin should be vertical.
- Extend the upper part of your elbow forward when hurling from mid-range to defend against counterattacks and maintain balance.

Curved Knee Techniques (Khao Khong)

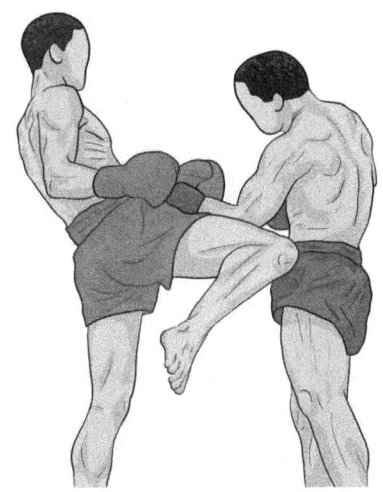

Khao Khong is effective in close combat.

Another excellent technique for beginners is the curved knee. This knee strike is particularly effective in close quarters, like tight clinches. This attack can be directed at your opponent's sides, specifically their hips, thighs, and ribs. Although this knee technique won't do as much damage to your opponent as others, it can be quite effective at slowing them down and depleting their energy.

Here are a few tips to help you get the better of your opponent using this technique:

- As you bend your knee into the object of attack, twist your hips.
- Move to the opposite side or gently slant your opponent's body.
- Ensure you have a firm footing when locked in the clinch position.
- Step back a bit before releasing your knee to your opponent's side.

Horizontal Knee Technique (Khao Tat)

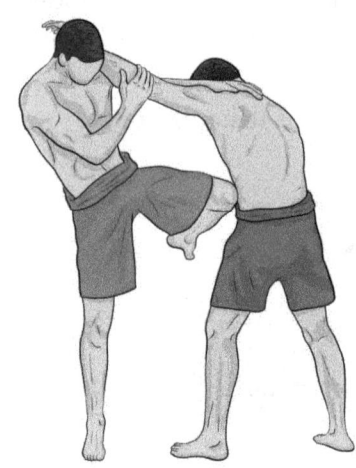

Khao Tat can be used offensively and defensively.

The horizontal knee technique is a common move among fighters, offensively and defensively. This knee technique can occasionally be a life-saver because it's quite simple to perform with the proper technique. Some fighters transition into a horizontal knee guard once they establish a connection with their opponent.

The horizontal knee is effective when launched from the back and the leading leg. The switch adds to this knee strike's diversity, especially in the clinch, as it can catch an opponent by surprise. Work hard on your balance and learn to establish an advantage over your opponent in the clinch while practicing this strike because, if not done correctly, you risk being swept off your standing leg.

Follow these tips when performing the Khao tat;
- Moving the striking leg upward parallel to the floor.
- Launch yourself forward, bending your shin into the object of your attack.
- Generate power by rotating and turning on the standing leg.

Diagonal Knee Techniques (Khao Chiang)

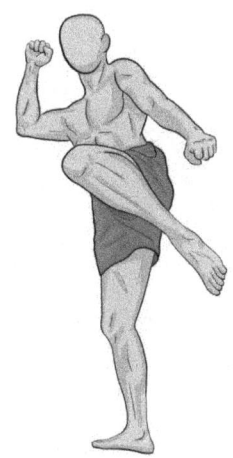

Khao Chiang is a short-range strike.

The diagonal knee is a second short-range strike that works inside and outside the clinch. It is targeted at your opponent's sides, especially the ribs. Its dynamics make it challenging to predict and, if executed well, could be a show-stopper. While coming from an open clinch to deliver the diagonal knee, do this:

- On your front foot, take a slight step back.
- Simultaneously move your striking leg forward.
- Flex your leg just enough so that the portion of your leg from the knee down is pointed at an upward 45-degree angle at the point of contact.

Flying Knee Technique (Khao Loi)

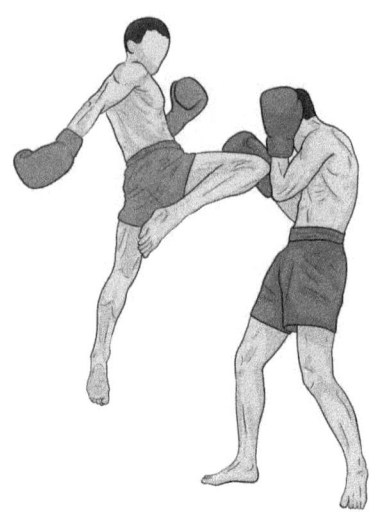

Khao Loi is a more advanced technique

Although this technique is far from what a beginner should concentrate on, it's okay to have an overview of how it works. To land this strike, you must have considerable technical skills and develop balance and posture. Still, you can do it with enough practice and commitment.

One of the hardest techniques to accomplish against an opponent in Muay Thai is to conceal a flying knee. This strike is quite effective when an opponent is unprepared. You might have witnessed some spectacular flying strike knockouts in MMA. Still, your chances of executing this technique in Muay Thai will most likely be restricted because fighters deliver this knee as a surprise attack against an opponent's attempt to take them down. Nevertheless, here is how to land a flying knee:

1. Ensure your opponent is in your line of sight.
2. While delivering the knee, fire upward, slightly bending your knees before driving up.
3. Twist the lead hip backward, then the opposite.
4. As you reach the top of your jump, extend your knee.
5. Lastly, protect your chin from counterattacks.

Small Knee Technique (Khao Noi)

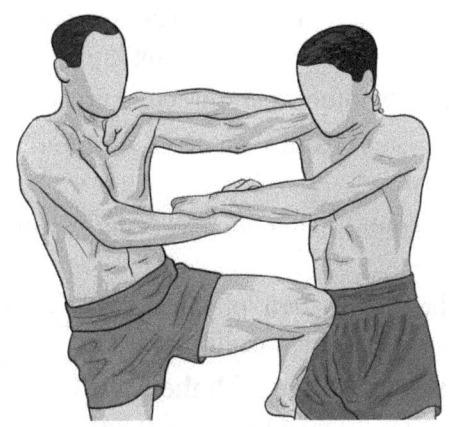

Khao Noican reduces your opponent's attacks.

In the clinch, the little knee is a powerful strike that can be executed. You can reduce your opponent's ability to move by delivering quick, little knees to their thighs. These can stop the opponent's momentum and lessen the force of their kicks and knees. An opponent with the advantage in the clinch might be persuaded to break off by the little knee strike, giving you time to change things up.

Long Knee Technique (Khao Yao)

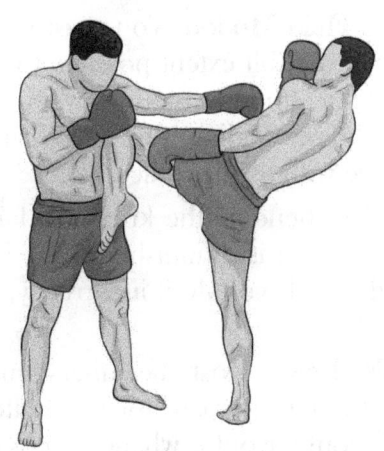

Khao Yao is effective from a long distance.

The long knee is the most effective strike from a great distance instead of a short range. It can potentially be an eye-catching spectacle because of the increase in impact with momentum. Your opponent might be unable to counter or defend against your attack, even if they anticipate the strike. Some ideas for the long knee include:

- Step out slightly rather than directly into your opponent
- Lift while twisting from your front foot and pressing your knee into the target
- Be certain your knee connects solidly with your opponent's body
- Pick up the pace when practicing this knee technique since throwing it is easier than drilling it slowly

Mistakes Made When Striking with the Knee

Following are some mistakes beginner fighters make while executing knee techniques.

Straightening Knee: While implementing the knee strike, you must understand that you're not trying to skim a person's body but to destabilize your opponent. Most beginners frequently thrust their knees straight up as if touching their adversary. Remember, you must penetrate through your opponent with your knee attack.

Although it is moving upward, you must attack your opponent's torso while aiming to breach your knees into them. Consider yourself at an angle, attempting to grab your opponent's ribs. In this situation, your kneecap should strike the opponent in the ribcage.

Failure to Achieve Fluid Motion: You must use your knee's strength, distance, and power to the full extent possible to perform a knee strike. You can only create a smooth motion when you mix these three components. Although extending the hips can be challenging for beginners, it is possible with regular practice.

Knee Not Bent: Not bending the knee is a fairly common error by novices. The strike's impact is diminished if the knee isn't bent since it isn't sufficiently solidified. If you do it incorrectly, you also risk suffering a major injury.

Dropping Hands Low: Most beginners make the mistake of positioning one hand low to prepare for a jab after a strike. It's not an excellent habit; you should avoid it whenever possible. Instead, lift both hands at once, defending your jaw from attack.

Launching Lunging from Afar: Beginners believe they can catch their opponent from a distance, like with a training bag. However, they soon discover their reach falls short as it exceeds the one they rehearsed with a bag. As a result, if you attempt to land the knee from the same distance during a fight, you'll fall short.

How to Strengthen and Condition the Knee for Strong Attacks

Although it takes time to build knee strength, you can hasten the process by learning the correct methods and exercises. Here are some guidelines to assist you in pulling it off.

Conditioning

No matter how skilled or gifted you are, it would all amount to nothing if you were not in shape. Sometimes you might be fortunate, but it will not be for long. You must ensure you are in the best condition to have strong knees. Every time you fight, you should be in top physical condition because you can bet your opponent will be.

A battery-operated torch comes to mind when discussing conditioning. When the batteries are juiced up, it becomes brighter; this applies to all fighters equally. Training is essential. Your legs, which you rely on for movement and striking in Muay Thai, will give out if they grow weary. As a beginner fighter, you must be in excellent shape since you depend on your legs. Here's how to improve your conditioning;

- Go for a 10-kilometer long-distance run five or more days a week.
- Do a series of sprints, like five rounds of 100m sprints in a row
- Go for mountain runs
- Do regular stretches and pushups
- Run up or take the stairs regularly.

The Right Team Coach and Coach

You will invariably improve your knee strikes with the correct coach and team. Before taking control of those knees, you must put much effort into your technique. Lifting weights or briefly carrying heavy objects over your head is not equivalent to producing energy in knee strikes.

Your technique must be perfected to produce the most power possible. Every part of a strike can be taken apart by a knowledgeable coach who will concentrate on how you stand, set up, execute, and deliver—practicing with fighters who will share a few suggestions here and there, is also essential.

Drills

Before adding power to your knee strike, you must first comprehend how crucial your stance, hips, feet, legs, and knees are for a great stroke. Each technique, the curved, straight, horizontal, or diagonal knee, must be practiced to develop power. In developing considerable power, the strike's fundamentals should be intuitive.

During the various training sessions, you must practice knee drills. Pick the knee strike you want to master, then spend as much time honing and repeating the drills required. Hitting your knees in sparring, on the bag, the pads, and during shadow boxing will help you develop your balance, positions, penetration, and timing. Your knee's strength can be increased by strengthening its vital parts. You will experience a change in the force you use to enforce the strike, albeit it might take a few weeks. You can get where you're going faster than you think if you pay careful attention to detail and focus appropriately.

How to Best Block a Knee When Fighting

If not correctly countered, Muay Thai knees can fracture the ribs. The following tips will help you defend against your opponent's knees, whether in or out of the clinch.

Extending your arm (jabbing) to your opponent's chest will block your opponent's knee if they are not in the clinch. Your arm should extend farther than your opponent's knee if you lean slightly into it. You should strike the chin as opposed to the chest.

When your opponent raises their leg to throw the knee while you are still engaged in the clinch, you can attempt to knock them off balance. Turn them in the direction of their standing leg. If they throw their right knee, you can turn to the right.

If the opponent shifts their weight beyond their standing leg, you can throw them or respond with your (right knee) knee. It takes some work to master this move because it is difficult to see your opponent's leg when engaged in the clinch. You must practice detecting it by observing how their weight changes.

The best offense is the best defense in Muay Thai. Therefore, as a Muay Thai fighter, it is essential to have effective techniques, understand how to produce power for your techniques, prevent common mistakes, and block your opponent's tactics. As a beginner, you should devote the same amount of effort to learning and practicing these knee techniques since they can truly be handy in emergencies. The best option for mastering the knee technique is a good training partner. You can strengthen each other's defenses and weaknesses, positioning yourself to be the best.

Chapter 6: Te: Kicking Techniques

Strong kicks are a significant part of Muay Thai. Being proficient in various kicking techniques allows you to develop powerful attacks, and they can also be very useful for defense. They help you keep your distance from the opponent, making it harder for them to reach you while still landing powerful blows to all areas of their body. Moreover, if you want to strike the opponent's legs, the most effective approach is to use good kicks.

Here are some of the most useful kicking techniques you should be well versed in and additional information to help you maximize your kicking techniques.

Top Kicking Techniques

These kicking techniques can be used on their own or combined. Depending on the situation and the attack you want to formulate, you can combine two kicks or pair some punches and upper-body moves with these kicks.

1. Spinning Round Kick – Tae Klap Lang

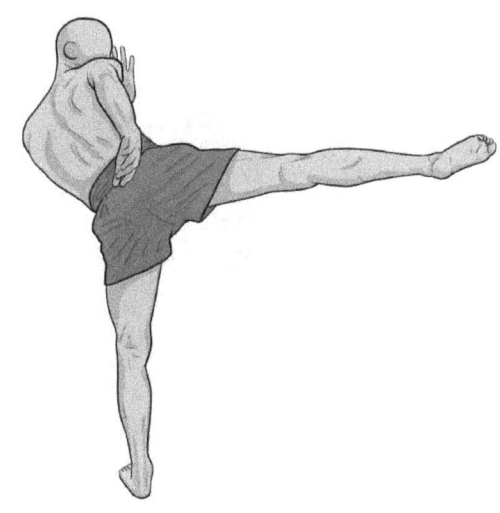

Tae Klap Lang is a powerful kick.

This kick is one of the most powerful kicks you can master. When used correctly, it can easily knock out your opponents; if used carelessly, it can be fatal. This kick is primarily used as a defensive strategy, but with the right combinations and setup, it can be part of your offensive strategy.

You will use your rear leg for this kick, creating a spinning motion. Your back faces the opponent, then spin your attacking leg around your body to create momentum. The target is the opponent's upper body, neck, and face.

It is the spinning motion that generates the momentum and what makes round kicks so deadly. For this kick, you should train your legs for flexibility and dexterity and work on hip mobility.

2. Jumping Push Kick – Kradot Teep

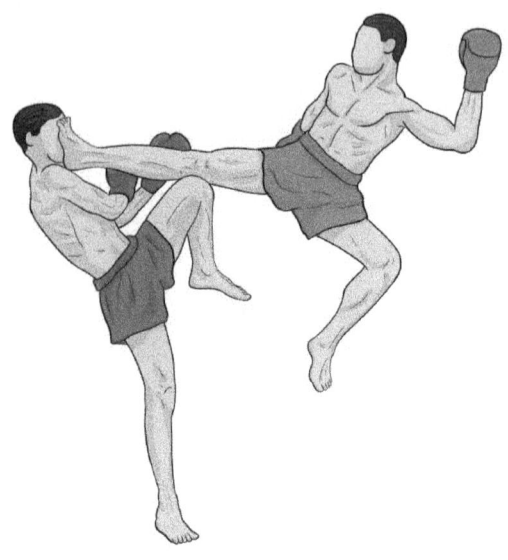

Kradot Teep will help you gain an advantage

If you don't have room to spin to create extra force in your kick or want to create more force in a kick while approaching an opponent, the jumping push kick will come in handy.

This kick is like the straight kick, except you use your rear leg to jump off the floor and create more momentum. A popular technique is to lead your opponent with your kicking leg, putting it straight up like you would with a straight kick but then jumping off your rear leg in the middle of the kick to generate extra force.

This kick is great for the upper body and face area. If you are going for the regular straight kick, it only takes a moment to transform it into the jumping push kick.

3. Straight Front Kick – Tae Trong

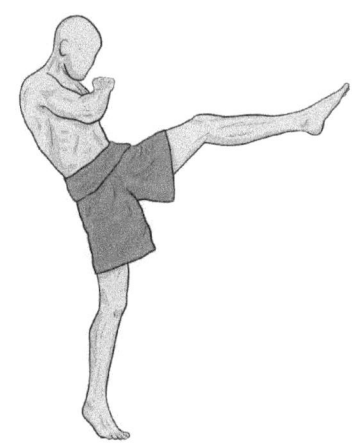

Tae Trong is similar to the Mae Geri Karate technique.

The straight front kick is commonly used in Karate. In Japanese, it is called *Mae Geri*.

With this kick, you use your toes or the upper part of your foot to attack the opponent instead of the sole of your foot. It is a simple forward kick aimed at the chin or the sides of the face.

4. Downward Roundhouse Kick – Tae Kod

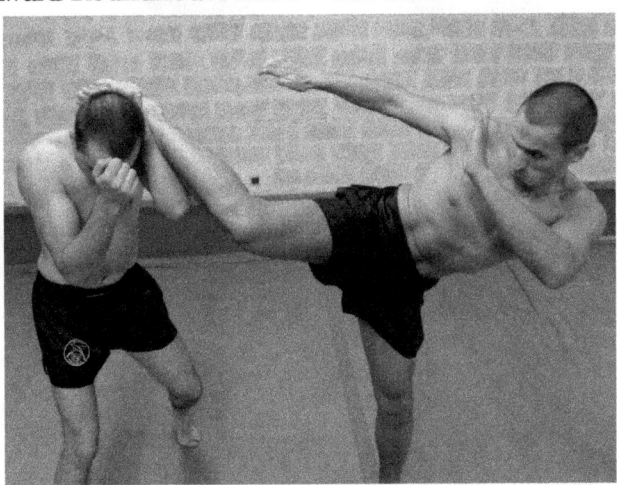

Tae Kod is known as the Brazilian Kick.
Krystof Gauthier (France), CC BY-SA 3.0 <https://creativecommons.org/licenses/by-sa/3.0>, via Wikimedia Commons: https://commons.wikimedia.org/wiki/File:Lethwei-Hight-kick.jpg

This kick is known as the question mark kick or the Brazilian kick. Again, due to the spinning motion required in the roundhouse movement, this kick generates a lot of momentum and can be devastating when used correctly.

The main difference from a traditional roundhouse kick is that your kicking leg has to be picked up higher in the downward roundhouse kick. Essentially, you must position your leg above your target, then angle your leg down onto the target to complete the move. It can be particularly challenging if your opponent is taller than you. Also, you must have excellent hip flexibility for this move as you spin around and push your leg upward.

This is an excellent kick as you nullify the opponent's guard and attack the head, neck, and shoulder area from above rather than from the front, where you would have to penetrate the guard.

5. Diagonal Kick - Tae Chiang

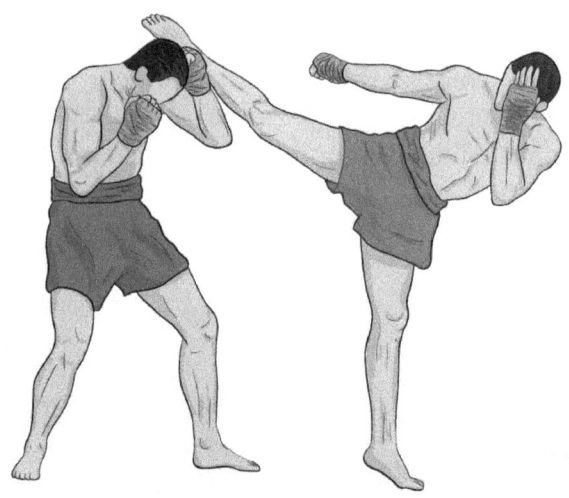

Tae Chiang is a quick kick.

This is a very quick kick using the shin to strike the opponent's body, specifically the ribs. This kick is perfect for close-quarter situations and can be a very painful blow when done right.

Typically, the attacker's leg has a 45-degree angle from the floor and is pushed straight into the opponent's sides.

6. Muay Thai Axe Kick – Tae Khao

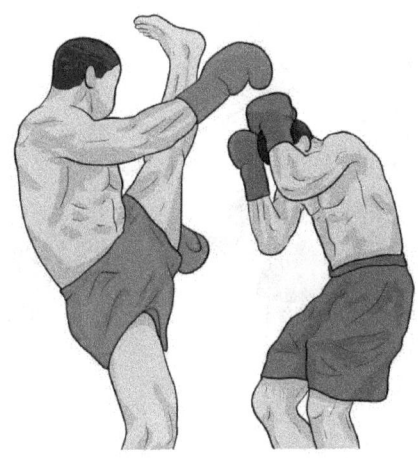

Tae Khao targets the face, neck, and shoulders

The Muay Thai axe kick is similar to the downward roundhouse kick but without the spinning movement to create momentum. This kick targets the face, neck, and shoulders.

From a standing position, the attacker launches a straight kick slightly above the target area, then drives the heel of the foot down onto the target area. Similar to an axe coming down on its target.

While this is a powerful kick, it opens the attacker to a quick counterattack, so fighters rarely use it.

7. Slapping Foot Thrust – Teep Top

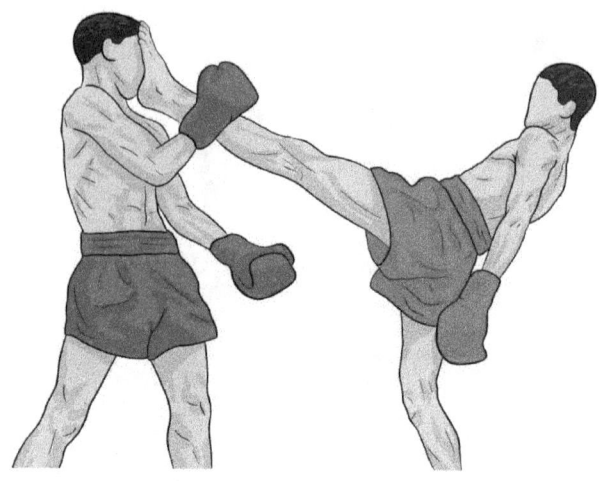

Teep Top is helpful for defense.

In this kick, the knee of the striking leg is bent, and the top of the foot or the entire foot is used to "slap" the opponent. Depending on how high you take your striking leg and whether you twist during this kick, it can be a straight kick to the abdomen, a slap to the ribs, or even a slap to the head.

This kick is a great move in a defensive situation. It helps keep the attacker off you and also unbalance the opponent. However, not much power can be generated from this kick.

8. Straight Foot Jab – Teep Trong

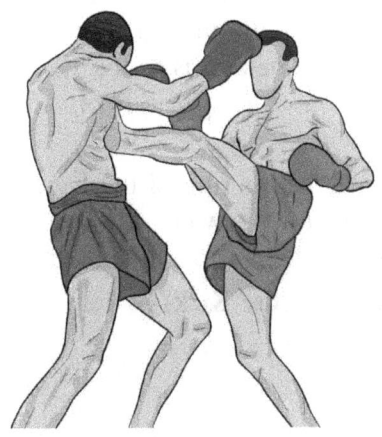

Teep Trong is usually aimed at the abdomen.

This quick, sharp, straight kick can be considered the leg version of a straight jab. For this move, you will lean back slightly and "punch" out in a straight line with your kicking leg. This kick is typically aimed at the abdomen and chest but can also be aimed at the head.

It is a great move for controlling the opponent's distance away from you. It can be used very effectively to push the opponent or unbalance them as they approach an attack. It can also be a good kick to unbalance your opponent before you launch your attack. These are considered blocking or "checking" kicks.

9. Muay Thai Side Kick – Te Tad

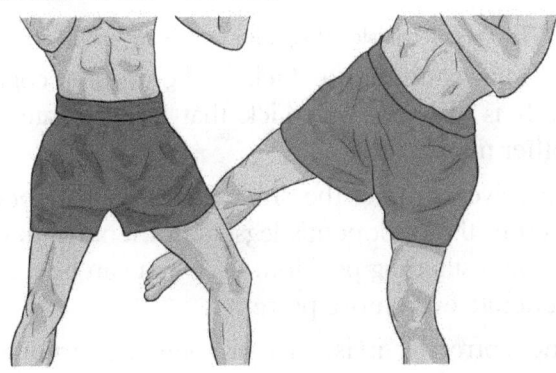

Te Tad is slightly different than a normal sidekick.

The sidekick in Muay Thai is slightly different than in other disciplines, such as Taekwondo and Karate. In Muay Thai, there is no chambering of the kicking leg. Rather, the fighter steps in with the standing leg to create momentum and then shoots out the kicking leg from the side of the hip. The aim is to hit the target with the sole of the foot, the side of the sole, or even the heel if the kick is aimed slightly higher at the chin or nose.

In other disciplines, chambering of the leg (pulling the knee into the chest) is used to generate power. However, this slows down the movement and opens the fighter to a counterattack.

10. Muay Thai Roundhouse Kick-Te Tat

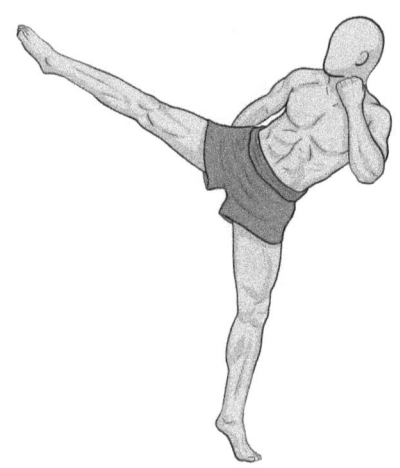

Te Tat differentiates Muay Thai from other martial arts.

The Muay Thai roundhouse kick is the most recognizable in this fighting form. It is also the one kick that differentiates a Muay Thai fighter from other martial artists.

This kick involves striking the shin against the opponent. This kick can be delivered to the opponent's legs, abdomen, head, or arms. It can be delivered from a standing position, or a spin can be incorporated into the move to generate even more power.

When done correctly, it is an extremely powerful and dangerous move. It can cause serious damage and even break tough bones, such as the opponent's shin or thigh bone.

Tips for the Roundhouse Kicks

The roundhouse kick is a very flexible and versatile kick to use in nearly any situation or purpose. Knowing how to execute this kick with the utmost precision will help you in countless situations.

Best Posture for Roundhouse Kicks

Before you launch your roundhouse kick, ensure you are in the right position. Firstly, your feet must be shoulder-width apart, with the bulk of your weight on the balls of your feet. You cannot drive power or accuracy into the kick if you aren't balanced when kicking.

The next most important thing to consider is your distance from the target. A good way to check is to throw a quick jab. If you can comfortably land a jab, you are at the right distance since the shin kick or knee kicks will be slightly longer range.

Lastly, you must have the right posture when launching the kick and throughout the movement. If you want to deliver a powerful kick, you must be balanced. Also, consider what the opponent can do in response to the kick; you should be positioned to handle any response.

You must focus on a few things to achieve a successful roundhouse kick. First, keep your weight on the ball of your foot when launching the kick and stay on the ball of your foot throughout the rotation. Ideally, you should spring up from the heel of your foot to the ball of your foot when you step in and launch the kick. This shift drives more power into the kick.

Also, ensure the foot of your pivoting leg is pointed out at a 45-degree angle when kicking. This will do two things; 1. You will have proper balance in the kick and, therefore, more power. 2. You will not be in the centerline of the kick so that you can negotiate a response from the opponent. Also, having your foot out at an angle decreases the distance your leg has to move, increasing the kick's perceived speed and power.

An open hip is an essential component of the roundhouse kick. It allows you to load the kick more effectively, gives better balance, facilitates better energy transfer, and drives momentum from your entire body into the kick. Moreover, it helps with stabilization after the kick, helping you spin back into position faster.

Common Mistakes

As discussed in the "best posture" section, the hip is crucial in the roundhouse kick and is often the one area where people make a mistake. Making this one mistake can lead to numerous problems. Ensuring your hip is open and your feet are in the right position will solve this issue.

Another issue is kicking with the foot; this is very common for people new to Muay Thai. Hitting something with your shin can hurt quite a bit, so it's important to condition your shins. However, during kicking training, you must focus on hitting the target with the center of your shin, where you have the most momentum.

Returning from the kick is another problem. Your leg must come back down to the ground just as fast as it went up with the roundhouse kick. Being slow in this part of the kick will put you in a vulnerable position where you can easily be taken down.

Another issue is timing the kick and having good defense during the kick. Even though it is powerful, the roundhouse kicks must be timed properly for the best results. You don't want to be caught by the opponent or be countered to the point where you are in trouble! Throwing a few punches or checking kicks, double-checking that you are off to one side of the opponent, and having good positioning with your arms to protect your chin will make a massive difference in how securely you land the roundhouse kick without being an easy target for the opponent.

Leg Conditioning

You need strong legs and shins to get proficient in the roundhouse kicks. You can do a few things for this:

The first is the heavy bag. Ideally, do 200 kicks on each leg on the heavy bag three times a week. It doesn't have to be very hard; even a soft bag will do. The idea is to deaden the nerves on the shin. Over time, as the nerves become less responsive to the kicks, they will stop hurting as much since they are no longer sending pain signals to your brain.

Next, do plenty of box jumps and squat jumps to help strengthen the tibia and fibula. Doing 5 sets of 15 of these exercises 2 or 3 times a week will condition your shin bones and prepare them for the heavy stress they face in the ring.

Lastly, you must do plenty of sparring with the shin pads on. Even with shin pads, heavy sparring has a massive impact on your shins. It will work wonders for strengthening and seasoning them to withstand high impact.

Blocking Kicks

To block a roundhouse kick, lift your shin and block in a shin-on-shin fashion. Lift your knee to a roughly 90-degree angle between your shin and thigh. Of course, if you block a kick to the midsection, your knee will be higher up. You can use your shin to block blows to the shins, thighs, and abdomen. You must use your arms for defense against anything coming to your chest or head.

The roundhouse kick is a fantastic kick to use in many situations. However, to make the most of it, you must know how to perform it correctly, avoid common mistakes, and have legs that are properly conditioned for this skill. Good leg training will help you land excellent kicks and give you protection for defending yourself from roundhouse kicks.

Chapter 7: Teep: Foot Techniques

Foot sweeps are important in Muay Thai. Whether sparring or competing at the highest level, having several different foot kicks and foot sweeps at your disposal will put you in a better position in combat.

While the sweep is simple, it can be applied in many ways to unbalance your opponent, disarm them from an attack, or set them up for your attack. Like many other things in Muay Thai, excellent foot technique is about speed and timing. Here is everything to know about the different foot techniques in Muay Thai.

Muay Thai Foot Kicks

Muay Thai foot kicks are important in a fight. They deflect oncoming attacks, unbalance the opponent, and also block or check kicks. These kicks are primarily targeted at the opponent's abdomen, chest, or face. Still, they can also be used on the legs and to defend against kicks. In these quick kicks, the toes, heel, or sole can be used to attack the opponent. These are also called "foot slaps" since they are less powerful than a straight kick or well-positioned punch. However, with speed and accuracy, you can use them to great effect.

There are two main forms of foot kicks, listed below.

1. Straight or Forward Foot Kick (Teep Trong)

From a standing position, the fighter lifts his knee and kicks out forward with his shin to land his foot on the opponent. Typically, this is used for attacking above the waistline. It is an excellent attack at the opponent's abdomen, chest, or face but must be executed quickly. The kick back to the body must be just as fast as the kick out to the opponent. Good hip mobility will also be required to use the teep trong for the face.

2. Sideways Foot Kick (Teep Khang)

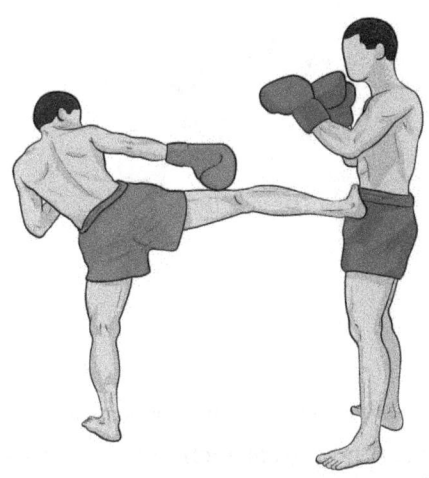

Teep Khang is used similarly to when a straight kick is used.

This kick is used in the same fashion as the straight kick. The difference is that the fighter is on their side when launching the attack. This way, the fighter's side faces his opponent, the hips are turned to the side and dipped down, facing the floor, and the side of the sole lands on the opponent. Since this move involves rotating the hips, it has a bit more force since momentum from the upper body is transferred into the kick. This kick is slightly more challenging as it requires better hip mobility and balance to be carried out properly. Foot position, hip rotation, and even how the upper body is positioned will influence how well one can balance in a teep khang.

Standing Foot Sweeps

Sweeps are used extensively in Muay Thai and can benefit the fighter. Several versions of sweeps can be employed, depending on the situation. This section covers some of the most basic but also most versatile sweeps you should master.

1. Catch and Sweep

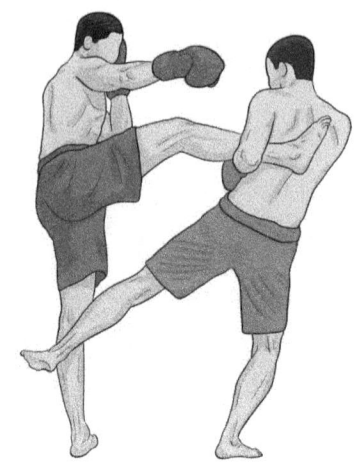

The catch and sweep is a great response to kicks.

The catch and sweep is a great technique used to amazing effect in response to kicks. It is one of those things most opponents will not expect. Usually, a checking kick is used to block kicks. The sweep will block the kick and make it less likely for the opponent to use that kick again since they know it will be viciously countered.

For this sweep, catch the sidekick or roundhouse kick with your arms, nearly hugging the leg as you catch it to minimize impact. Next, lift the opponent's leg slightly and switch your steps. This will unbalance the opponent and make sweeping them off their feet easier. As your opponent tries to hop to regain balance, you can very easily sweep them down to the canvas with a kick to the calf of their pivoting leg.

2. Roundhouse Sweep

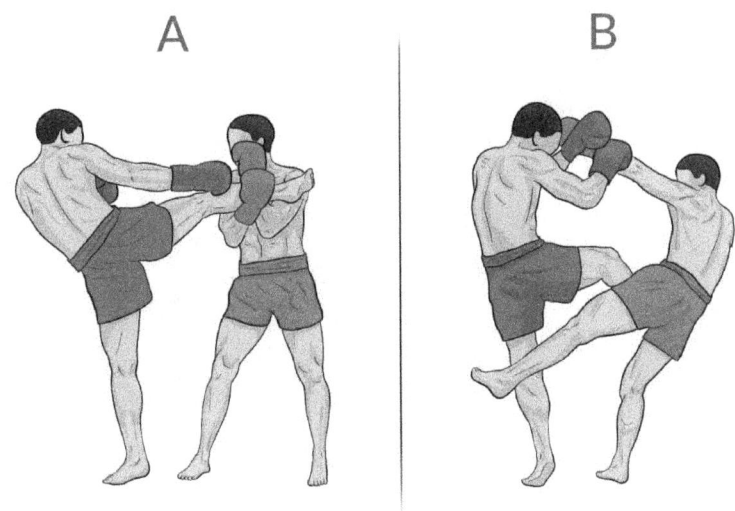

The roundhouse sweep can allow you so exploit your opponent.

This sweep exploits the tendency of most fighters to respond to a kick with a kick. If you throw a roundhouse kick to your opponent, you can be nearly certain they will throw one back.

For this sweep, throw a roundhouse kick to the body to see how your opponent reacts. If you get a kickback from them, throw another one to prime them for the sweep. These initial kicks are to prep the opponent. Putting too much force into them is unnecessary as you risk being caught and countered.

Before the opponent can reply with their second kick, use your rear leg, targeting the ankle area on the opponent's rear leg to kick them off balance while their lead leg is in the air for an attack. Ideally, you want to land your sweep blow while the opponent's attack leg is in the air. This way, you can ensure their weight is on their leg, and the sweep will be effective. Depending on your opponent's height and reach, this might require you to take a small step forward.

3. Rear Sweep

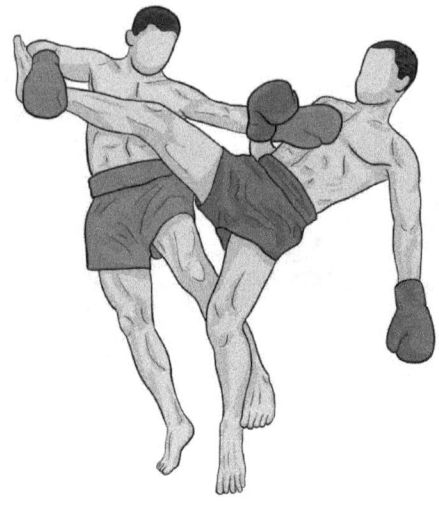

The rear sweep can be painful for your opponent.

This is a great sweep and quite painful for the opponent since they land completely flat on their body when all their weight is involved. This sweep is best done after a few punches or kicks to be sure your opponent is putting the bulk of their weight on the rear leg.

As you kick the right side of the opponent's body, they will put up their right leg to defend. On the second or third kick, throw a feint kick to the right and move in with your rear leg to sweep the leg they are standing on. For an even better effect, use your opposite hand to move their leg out of the way to get closer and push them back on their pivoting leg so all their weight is on the leg you are about to sweep.

4. Teep Counter Sweep

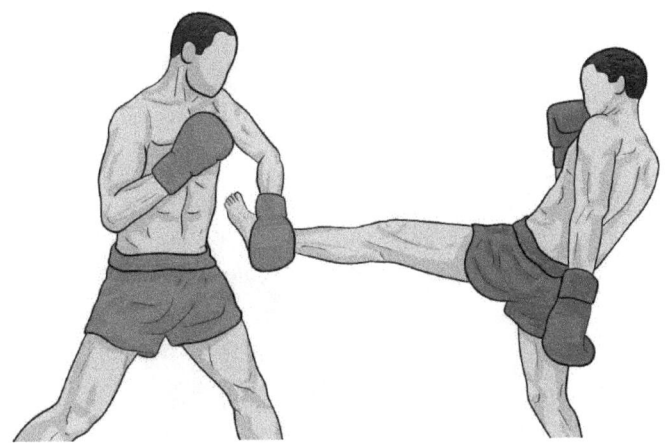

The teep counter sweep is a valuable skill

One of the most common attacks you will encounter is the forward teep. Knowing how to counter this attack with a quick and effective sweep is a valuable skill.

The objective is to catch the opponent's leg during a teep, pull them towards you, take out their pivoting leg, and push them down as they fall for greater impact against the canvas.

Ideally, catch their leg in a vice grip cupping the back of their ankle with one hand. Then, jerk them toward you to unbalance them and bring their pivoting leg into range. Next, kick their pivoting leg in the ankle area to execute the sweep and finish with a strong push to the chest or shoulders to speed up the fall and increase impact against the canvas.

5. Low Kick Feint to Sweep

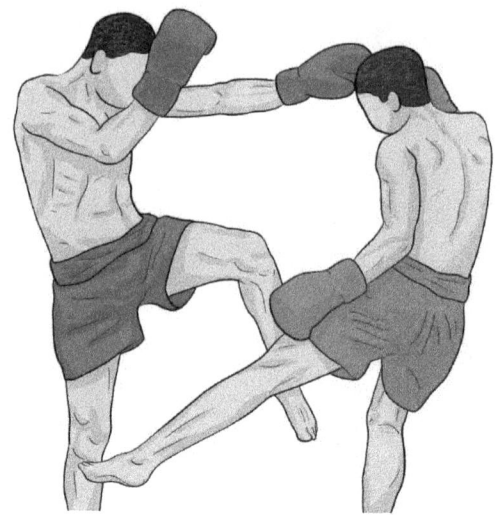

The low kick feint to sweep can help you brock your opponent's attacks.

The objective is to sweep under your opponent's rear thigh to get them on the canvas. Again, you must set up your opponent with a few low kicks or kicks to the ribs to get them in the right position to execute your sweep.

Move in close to your opponent as they lift their leg to defend against what looks like a kick. As their leg is up in the air and all their weight is on the pivoting leg, throw a hard kick to the inner side of their rear thigh to get them to land flat on the floor. Having your hand out in front of you with your chin secured behind your shoulder is also a good approach so you are ready to block any oncoming counters.

If you want to increase the impact, push the opponent as they begin to fall to increase the speed of the fall.

Benefits of Foot Sweeps

Sweeps are commonly used in many martial arts. Each martial art has certain sweeps unique to that particular martial art. Also, many sweeps might be allowed in one martial art but not in other martial arts in a competitive setting.

Having multiple sweeps at your disposal as a Muay Thai athlete would be a good idea. Here are some of the main benefits a sweep provides:

Strike Setup

Sweeps are an excellent way to unbalance your opponent. When learning to sweep, there will be many instances where you don't do a clean sweep, but even then, you will have displaced your opponent. This moment of instability is all you need to launch a full attack and possibly end the match.

If you are using Muay Thai as part of your MMA training, where ground and pound are permitted, then sweeps are a useful technique to get the opponent on the floor. Moreover, when an opponent lands hard on the floor in a sweep, it is tough for them to stabilize and be prepared for the groundwork required to fight on the ground. In both cases, you benefit from the sweep.

Match Pace

A player's rhythm is significant in their match performance, especially if the player can synchronize their moves with footwork and a natural fighting rhythm. You can use the sweeps to disrupt this rhythm effectively. When you sweep an opponent, it takes them a moment to get back up and restart their rhythm. Doing this enough times and with enough force during a match can be devastating for the opponents' rhythm. A lack of rhythm leads to bad timing, causing poor impact and making it harder for them to dodge and defend your attacks.

Sweeps have much more impact than just a plain kick or punch to the body. If you want to tire your opponent, break their confidence, and hurt their body, then sweeps will be more effective than quick kicks and jabs. Moreover, when you add a hard push to a sweep, it is even more dangerous.

Space

Regardless of how seasoned you are, going head-to-head with a strong opponent can be tiring. Sweeps are a great way to earn you a few moments to take a few deep breaths and refresh yourself. If your opponent is constantly on you, it makes it hard to breathe and focus; sweeps will earn you some space to gather yourself. If you're ever in a tight situation, throwing a sweep will help give you some clarity.

Dominance

The mind game, especially your frame of mind, plays a major role in your fight performance. Sweeps are one of those moves that give you confidence while demotivating your opponent. It gives you a moment to think; when you are more confident, you can formulate better plans.

Standing tall above your opponent after a sweep influences your psychology directly and subconsciously. If you feel you cannot land anything on your opponent but then successfully break out a sweep, it can drastically change the situation. Moreover, being on the mat flat on your back in competition chips away at a player's confidence. Falling down and getting back up tires out a fighter - another added benefit of sweeps.

Points

It's not always about hurting your opponent. In a competition setting, the objective is to score points, and sweeps can earn valuable points with the judges. It also shows the judges that you control the situation and have excellent spatial awareness.

Sweeps can stop your opponent from scoring too many easy points with small, quick moves. If you feel a round is getting out of your control, throwing a sweep will help level things for the next few seconds.

Illegal Sweeps

Knowing the illegal sweeps, especially for players coming from other martial arts, is important. Players coming from Taekwondo, Jiu-Jitsu, and Judo have the most problems in this regard. Common sweeps in those sports, such as Ouchi Gari and Ostoro Gari, are illegal in Muay Thai. *All sweeps involving picking up the opponent from the waist or using a limb are also illegal in Muay Thai.*

Knowing sweeps is crucial, but it takes time and practice to perfect the art of implementing a good sweep at the right moment to turn the tables. It takes a lot of practice to anticipate moves and engineer the appropriate sweep for the situation. Further sections explore how to pair sweeps with other moves to create combinations to overcome your opponent.

Chapter 8: Chap Kho: Clinching and Neck Wrestling Techniques

Perhaps the most iconic aspect of Muay Thai, besides the Mangkon, is the clinching and neck wrestling moves fighters use. In Western-style boxing and even some martial arts forms, clinching is not allowed. If two fighters get in a clinch, they are instantly broken up, or the fight is paused. Fighters in other combat sports, especially Western-style boxing, use clinching to defend themselves from oncoming attacks and to get a little break during the fight.

In Muay Thai, clinching is an essential part of the fight. It is one of the most intense and dangerous situations a fighter can be in. With the right skills and approach to clinching, it can be a game-changing skill for a fighter who knows what to do in a game. Fighters who favor the Muay Plam technique are all about clinching, just as Muay Sok is all about elbows; Muay Thai is about kicks. If you want to specialize in Muay Plam, or you merely want to improve your clinching game, this chapter covers everything to know.

Most Common Clinching Techniques

Different clenching techniques can be used to set up your opponent, defend, sweep, kick, knee, or other objectives. Some of the most commonly used and versatile techniques are the following:

1. Double Collar Tie

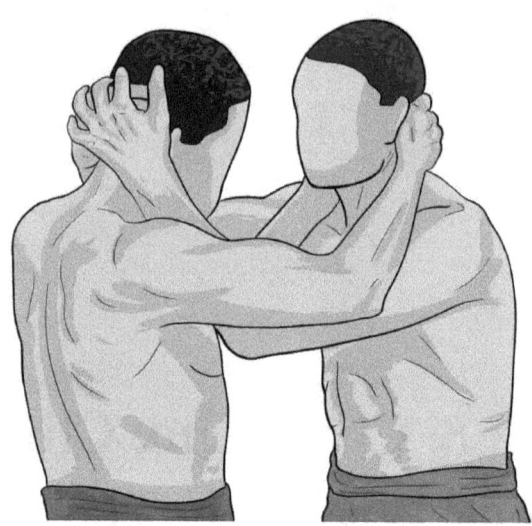

The double collar tie is a common clinching technique.

This technique is one of the most common clinching techniques in Muay Thai. It has been used by many of the best in the sport to amazing effect, including the highly decorated Petchboonchu. This technique is a favorite of knee-style fighters as it allows excellent control over opponents and opens their heads and abdomens to knee attacks.

There are two versions of the double collar tie; around the head or the neck.

If your objective is getting to the head, start by getting your hand through their guard and around the back of their head. Then, take the second hand and follow a similar path so you have both hands behind the opponent's head. From this position, it is very easy to bring the head downward for a blow with the elbow or knee. Also, maneuvering the body is far easier once you have good control of the head. You can easily set up the opponent's body for knee shots to the sternum and abs. In this grip, it's easier to spin the opponent around and move their body if you want to set them up for other attacks.

The other option is to grab the opponent's neck. For this, get your hands around the back of their neck and use a gable grip to clasp your hands together. This particular grip gives you excellent control, making it harder for the opponent to break your grip and allowing you to squeeze their neck. With this grip, it can be quite painful when you close your forearms into the sides of their neck, making this grip effective. You won't have as much control over their body from this position, but it is still an effective clinch in many situations. This will be particularly useful for opponents a bit taller than yourself. Reaching for their head will expose your abdomen, which can be extremely risky. However, by grabbing their neck, you are protecting yourself while also bringing yourself into striking range of the opponent.

2. Single Collar Tie

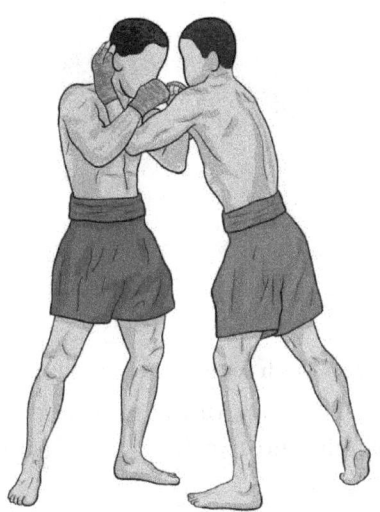

The single-collar tie is more commonly practiced.

The double-collar tie can certainly lead your opponent into a lot of damage. However, it is relatively easy to defend against and not that difficult to break once you understand how to counter it. The single-collar tie is a more commonly practiced clinch for these reasons.

This technique involves having one hand around the opponent's neck while the other hand is wrapped tightly against the opponent's bicep on the opposite side. With your right hand around the opponent's neck, your left hand should firmly grasp the opponent's right bicep. This way, you have good control over their entire body since there are two places where you can move their weight and unbalance them. Moreover, this clinch is more challenging to break, and while you can't hit the head easily from this position, you still have plenty of opportunity to knee their abdomen and chest and throw them around.

In this position, you can use your left hand (the one on the bicep) to land heavy uppercuts and hooks to the opponent's face. As you gain more experience in this position, you will learn to throw hard elbows using your right hand to the opponent's face and chest.

3. Over-Under Clinch Position

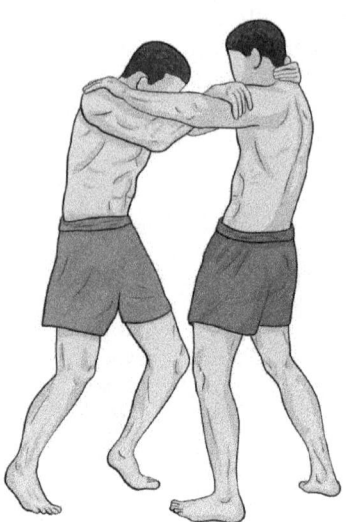

The over-under clinch position is very common in Muay Thai.

The over-under clinch is one of the most common clinch positions in Muay Thai. It is versatile and can be used effectively if you understand how it works.

In this position, you will have one arm coming over your opponent's arm with your hand on their neck while your other arm snakes under their opposite arm. Depending on your reach length, both hands could be on the opponent's neck, or one will reach their shoulder or bicep. In either case, with a good grip, you can do plenty of maneuvers from this position.

You can use your upper arm to pull your opponent down and your lower arm to push them up. If you have a longer reach, you can reach around your opponent and clasp your hands together in a tight hug to gain more control of the situation.

In this clinch, you can use your knees effectively into the opponent's sides or abdomen and are in a good position to deflect oncoming knee attacks. It is easy to push and pull the opponents to unbalance them and even sweep them down onto the mat. However, due to the close range, being proficient in defense in this position takes a lot of practice and fight awareness.

4. Double Underhooks

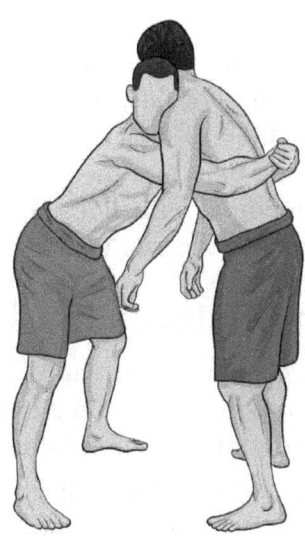

The double underhook is a common clinch in combat sports.

This is a common clinch in Western wrestling, MMA, Judo, and other combat sports involving ground fighting. In Muay Thai, ground fighting is close to non-existent. However, this clinch can still be used effectively for unbalancing the opponent and gaining control of the situation. Moreover, its close proximity also protects you and acts as a form of defense from knees, albeit your sides will still be exposed, so be ready to react. If you want to carry out sweeps, this is also a great clinch to use for this purpose. This grip gives a good stance to generate power and enough reach to sweep your opponent even when both their feet are on the mat.

To get into this clinch, scoop your hands under the opponent's arms and reach around to their back. Your arms should go down under their arms, through the bottom of their shoulders, and around their back. You can clasp your hands behind their back if you can reach that far. Simultaneously, move your hips forward to nearly touch the opponent's. The closer your hips are to the opponent, the more control you will have since your body weight is significant rather than only your upper body strength.

The tricky thing about this clinch is getting too carried away with shoving your opponent and shuffling around on your feet. Moving too much will move your center off balance, and your opponent can easily use this to their advantage. The objective is to counter the opponent's moves with opposite moves while moving your body weight in the opposite direction.

Once you have mastered the basics, you can use this clinch to bump, lift, and swivel your opponent. For this, your hands must be lower down on their back, around the base of their ribs, from where you can get a tighter lock around them and then pick them up, bump into them, swivel them around, and throw them onto the floor. Managing your opponents' weight from this position makes it easier to sweep in many ways.

Common Mistakes in Clinching

Developing good clinch technique is one part of the clinching game. You must perfect many other aspects of clinching to dominate this style and phase of the fight. Here are some common issues to consider:

Stance - Many fighters walk into the clinch with their regular fight stance; this leads to a weak clinch and exposes you to several attack possibilities. The clinch stance is distinctly different from your regular fight stance. Ensure you don't mix the two and make the change at the right time. How smoothly you can transition into the clinch stance will play a big role in how effective you are in the clinch.

Knee Impact - Getting into the clinch is one thing, but making the most of the clinch boils down to how effectively you can knee your opponent. Initially, your knees will not have much impact, leaving the opponent thinking you are just tapping them with your knees. While you might feel you are driving a lot of force into the knees. It takes practice to deliver a painful knee to the abdomen.

This technique requires much practice on the heavy bag. Practice driving the point of your knee into the opponent. When kneeing the sides, ensure you drive the hard knee bone into the opponent, not just push your knee against their side. With low knee impact, your clinch technique is of little use.

Open Neck - The clinch is all about getting the neck or the head. Many fighters leave their neck completely exposed when going into the clinch, giving their opponent easy access and, consequently, easy access to controlling the clinch. Ensure your defense is up when going into the clinch, making it as hard as possible for your neck or head to be given away. Fight back and resist if you sense that your opponent is going for the neck. You can always break free and go in again, so you get to their neck first.

Wrestle – The clinch is difficult to negotiate, especially when fighting a taller or stronger opponent. However, the objective of the clinch is not to overpower your opponent through your wrestling skills; it is a place to show what you can do with your knees and possibly your elbows and fists. Use the close-quarter situation to inflict damage, not to move your opponent around.

Transition Defense – Fighters will have good defensive posture, but as soon as it is time to clinch, their arms drop, or their head comes up to get into the clinch. This gives the opponent easy access to your body, and a blow from that close can easily be a knockout. You must maintain good defensive posture until the last moment you are about to grab the opponent.

Optimizing the Clinch

Here are a few tips to help you take your clinch game to the next level:

Damage Posture – Once you have your opponent in a clinch, keep them in a forward posture as long as you can. The only way for them to defend against their knees is to regain their upright posture, and the longer you can prevent them from doing so, the longer you can maintain control of the situation and land your blows.

Protect Your Neck – As long as you don't give your head or neck to your opponent, you control the clinch. The harder you make it for them to grab onto you in the clinch, the lower your chances of getting hit or thrown around.

Flexibility – There are multiple ways to attack while in the clinch. If you can't get your knees in, try elbows, punches, throwing your opponent, or anything else that works. Stay aware of the situation and be flexible to different attack options, depending on the circumstances. Land anything you can, as long as it is accurate.

The clinch is something most fighters prefer not to get involved in. However, if you can master the basics of the clinch and understand how to negotiate the situation, you can use it to your advantage. Especially if you are caught up with someone who isn't very good in the clinch, this can be your opportunity to pull the match in your favor.

Chapter 9: Combination Techniques

Muay Thai is a fast-paced sport with room for hard-hitting blows and intricate combinations that will leave the opponent stumbling. As a Muay Thai fighter, you must develop competence in both aspects of the fight. You need laser-sharp accuracy in your kicks, punches, and elbows, and you want them to land hard.

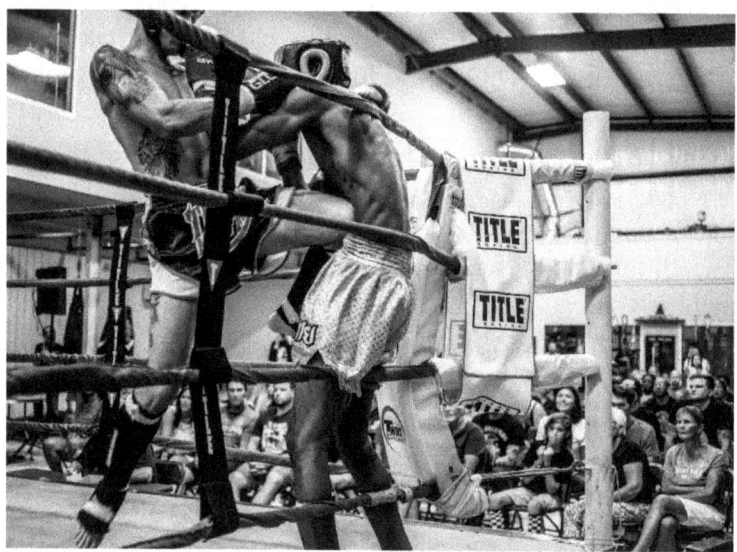

Muay Thai is a fast-paced sport.
https://unsplash.com/photos/1jaXXVuPRDc?utm_source=unsplash&utm_medium=referral&utm_content=creditShareLink

You also want to use these in different combinations to gain the upper hand in a match. This chapter looks at some of the best combinations to ensure a win.

Combinations

When using combinations, gauging distance before launching the combination and keeping track of where you are during the combination is vital. Sometimes, you might need to step forward during the combination, like throwing the combination while walking into the opponent. In other cases, it could be the opposite.

Also, be aware of how the opponent responds to the combination. It will not always be possible to land the entire combination, and in some cases, you must have room to add more moves to the combinations.

1. Fake Push Kick – Left Hook – Right Low Kick
1. First, fake a push kick to set up the opponent for this attack. This will give you the space and show you what to expect in the opponent's response to a push kick.
2. Nine out of 10 times, the opponent will raise a leg to defend against the oncoming kick. Here you want to take them by surprise and throw your left hook.
3. After the hook has connected, follow through with a strong kick to the opponent's lead leg or abdomen, depending on what is more easily accessible considering their defense and reaction.
4. If you manage to land all three, it will definitely have your opponent seeing stars. However, the key to this attack is deception. This combination will be more challenging against fighters familiar with your particular deception style and also with players who pick up deception quickly.

2. Jab – Overhand Right – Liver Kick
1. For this combination, start with a quick jab using your lead hand. This serves two functions. One is to get your opponent facing the direction of the jab. The other is to open them up for the rest of the attack.
2. Follow up the jab with a punch using your rear hand. It will be the punch that really has an impact, as you have a full range of motion to deliver this second punch.

3. In quick succession, deliver your kick (from the leg opposite the punching arm) to their midsection, ideally the liver. When you hit with your second punch, the opponent will raise their hands to defend, giving your kick access to the liver. However, you must be quick to make the most of this opportunity.

4. This combination incorporates hits to the upper and lower body making it hard to defend against, confusing, and also quite painful when done right.

3. Left Knee – Right Elbow – Left Hook

1. This combination starts with the left knee. To make this more effective, you can feint the opponent with a right leg kick to open them up and then step forward to get your left knee into their midsection.

2. Bring your left knee back down as soon as possible and shift your weight to the right, from where you throw your right elbow. You should aim for the temple, nose, jaw, or collarbone with your elbow.

3. Again, switch your weight to the opposite side, and while your opponent has their hands defending the right side, you come in with a swinging left hook.

4. This combination is about attacking from opposite sides with speed, not giving your opponent enough time to set up the necessary defenses. You will need good accuracy in your shots and excellent balance to carry this out properly.

5. If your opponent cannot handle this attack, continue with another elbow from the right and then back to the left knee to restart the loop.

4. Push Kick – Hook – Cross

1. Start with a push kick (teep) to get your opponent a step or two away from you and off balance. The added distance will help you take a step forward, adding momentum to the punch and allowing you to take a full swing.

2. Come in with a strong hook to the side of the head. Ideally, you want to target the temple, but anything on the side of the head will do.

3. Immediately after the hook, center your weight and come straight through the guard with a cross to the nose or chin.

4. For maximum effect, you must be lightning-quick after the teep to capitalize on the imbalance created by the push-kick.

5. Jab – Cross – High Kick

1. Start the attack with a jab. This will inflict some damage, but more importantly, it will distract the opponent.
2. Immediately, come through with a strong cross from the opposite end. Here you must make as much impact as possible.
3. Next, launch the high kick to the face, neck, or collarbone area. Generally, a straight kick will be the quickest option, but if you are exceptionally fast, you could squeeze in a roundhouse kick. In either case, the element of surprise is the highlight of this combination.

6. Jab – Cross – Left Hook – Right Knee

1. Start with a quick jab to see how your opponent reacts and to create some room in the center for your next move.
2. In nearly the same movement as the first jab, release a cross straight through their guard. You want to make the most of the moment when they are distracted by the jab.
3. Again, in quick succession, throw in the left hook while they are recovering from the cross and putting up their gloves in front of their face anticipating another blow but leaving the sides of their face open.
4. Lastly, throw in a strong right knee to the midsection. If you have the opportunity, grab the opponent to ensure they stay in position to receive the knee.

7. Jab-Cross-Switch Kick

1. Here, you use a quick jab to "open up" the attack.
2. As soon as your opponent starts to defend potential hooks, put a cross straight through their guard. You will temporarily unbalance them, making it harder for them to focus on what to defend next.
3. At this point, switch your feet so your lead foot falls back. You want to swing your rear leg out using the momentum you developed from the switch foot technique and aim for the opponent's neck or head. With more room, you will easily swing high and, with a full swinging motion, drive immense

force into the kick.

8. Left Elbow – Straight Right – Left Uppercut

1. Getting an elbow on your opponent can be a game-changer. Even if you don't land it with 100% accuracy, it can still do a lot of damage. In this combination, start with a left elbow to the opponent's face, neck, or collarbone.

2. It will be enough to put them off balance as a lot of body weight is behind an elbow. With the opponent unbalanced and their guard out of place from the elbow, you create the opportunity to launch a straight right. Ideally, you should do this with the same arm you landed the elbow with. Do this without pulling your elbow back but driving a straight punch in that small area.

3. By this time, you have opened up a good size cavity. Here you can capitalize on the opportunity and use your left arm again for an uppercut or a blow to the solar plexus.

This in-the-face combination is best suited to fighters comfortable in close-range situations. However, it is an excellent combination for others to practice against the pads or the bag to help with speed. It will improve fluidity in your moves in those tight spaces and make the most of your available space.

9. Push Kick – Cross – Left Hook – Right Knee

1. Again, the evergreen Teep (push kick) will come into play. Start the combination by pushing your opponent back and getting them off balance.

2. Quickly moving forward to catch up with your opponent, follow up with a cross straight into your opponent.

3. A left hook to the side of the head should closely follow the cross,

4. Next, bring the right knee to the opponent's midsection with as much impact as possible. Again, you can grab onto the bicep or the neck to hold your opponent in position while you drive in a knee.

This combination is a comprehensive attack that can yield excellent results, but it takes practice to execute properly. It is a combination requiring a higher degree of coordination and also stamina. Practice this thoroughly until you can execute it flawlessly before using it in a game. You don't want to get caught up in the middle of your combination with a counterattack.

10. Right Cross – Left Uppercut – Right Roundhouse Kick

1. This is another combination that starts with a punch to the face. To make this possible, you must look for the right opening to successfully land a good cross to the opponent's nose, cheek, or chin.
2. A good cross will disorient your opponent, giving you the room to proceed with the next step, a left uppercut. If you can connect this left uppercut to the opponent's chin, it will certainly have them walking around with wobbly legs.
3. The last piece of the puzzle is the roundhouse kick. As you land your uppercut, pivot your weight on your lead foot, shifting the momentum to the other side, where you can launch a heavy roundhouse kick to the opponent's body or head.

The main element of this combination is the roundhouse kick at the end, hopefully leading to a knockout win. However, you must be on point with the punches to get it done right. It is the punches that will put the opponent in the right position to deliver the roundhouse kick easily without the issue of being blocked or countered.

What determines how effective a combination will be is the timing with which you launch it. One strategy is to look for the perfect moment to launch a combination that will last the entire length. The other approach is to attack whenever you see a slight opening and go as far as possible with the combination. You can never be certain how your opponent will react, so it's best to make the most of every chance and inflict as much damage (score as many points) as possible in every burst.

These are some of the best combinations in a Muay Thai faceoff. However, remember, in a competitive environment; there are rules you must stick to. There are other ways of executing these combinations and many ways to make them more lethal – but always stay within the confines of the regulations when competing.

Also, regardless of how good you are at the combinations, you must be proficient in managing your opponent's weight in the ring. The power you develop for these combinations will come from the momentum you get through weight distribution and channeling your weight to the side you attack from. When you can better control your opponent's weight, you can use this to your advantage to create more momentum in your attacks. Practice these combinations on pads and bags, but also during sparring. It will give you the real-fight experience of managing yourself and your opponent.

Chapter 10: Defense Tips and Techniques

Muay Thai is a dangerous martial art with techniques that can be used as a defense in the ring, on the street, and outside. This combat style is known worldwide as the "deadly art of 8 limbs," which uses kicks, knees, elbows, punches, clinch movements, etc. Its origin is as far back as the old South-Asian kickboxing era. As a Muay Thai fighter, it is not enough to learn better ways to strike or attack your opponent; a defensive position is as necessary as an offense.

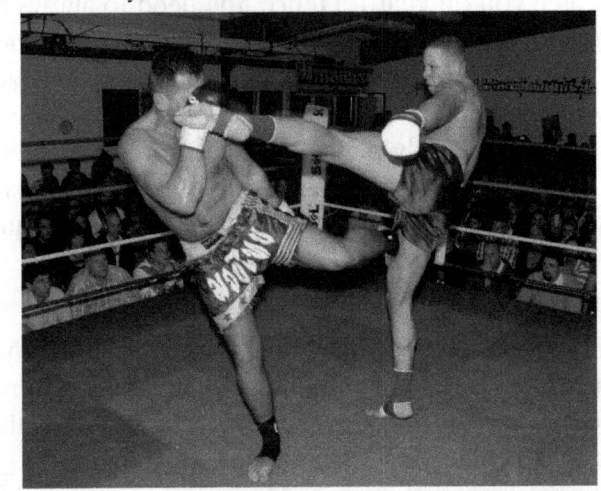

Muay Thai is a sport that requires you to be able to defend yourself.
https://commons.wikimedia.org/wiki/File:USMC-081025-M-0884D-005.jpg

This chapter teaches the many ways to block a strike and give a counter-attack in any position, in the ring or the street, and the essential tools to master for a good defense anytime, anywhere.

Muay Thai directs your focus on a simple yet effective strike position, using several limbs to attack or quickly defend against an attack. These are done in a matter of seconds, so as a fighter, you must build short-term focus and speed to have a great advantage in the world of Thailand kickboxing. As you journey through the defense tips and techniques for Muay Thai, get your mind ready to be exposed to the fundamentals, the benefits of good defense techniques, and practical ways to defend and remain dominant in the ring and on the street.

Fundamentals of a Good Defense

Unlike most combat sports, many factors must be considered when participating in Muay Thai. You must learn fundamental skills to build good defense techniques. These techniques might seem difficult to beginners, but remember that even world-class professionals had difficulties when they first trained. So, do not get overwhelmed and discouraged on your journey; follow the tips below to build a good defense in this combat sport:

Having a Tight Guard

In combat, you get all these limb attacks coming from every angle, and they can catch you off guard. Hence, the need to always be guarded. When your guard is tight, it will be hard for your opponent to land punches and strikes on sensitive areas like your face or head. It is also advised that while keeping a tight guard, you should ensure it is flexible enough to protect other body parts. The reason is the flexibility of your guard makes it easy to see or predict your opponent's next move and block or defend the strike. It is an essential skill to be equipped with when using Muay Thai techniques.

Movement of Your Head

Knowing how to move your head and dodge punches is useful when facing head-to-head with an opponent that lands many punches. Unpredictable head movements are not only for boxers, as they can also be applied in a sport like Muay Thai. Head movement is a great way to avoid strikes to the face. Although in Muay Thai, you should know that ducking under punches is a terrible way to defend and prevent them. You will likely get a knee kick in the face if you do. This is not to override the need to dodge punches, just a call to caution not to exaggerate certain head movements to avoid your opponent gaining an advantage.

Balance

In the art of self-defense, balance is a crucial factor that must be deliberated. When your defense style is a firm stand but adventurous, you could get kicked in the face and set off guard. If your legs aren't firm on the ground, you will be thrown off balance, giving your opponent an upper hand. So, how can you imbibe this? Take a stance that keeps you on your feet, even with several shots. Keep the space between your feet wide enough to give good stamina. You won't easily stumble over after you get kicked or punched when you do this.

Calculated Movement

Accuracy is paramount to getting a cool and perfect shot on your opponent. A well-calculated move would stun your opponent and make them double-check their next move. For example, elbows are an important move, but with the right timing and distance, it could knock your opponent out. Elbows and kicks are Muay Thai combat's most dangerous and powerful techniques.

Benefits of Muay Thai Defense

In every combat style outside of Muay Thai, defense and offense are common topics that are never overlooked. Although other combat styles have good defense and offense techniques, none surpasses those in Muay Thai. Thailand kickboxing allows you to blend as many techniques as you can. Due to its practicality and flexibility, and uses of all body limbs, you can learn several techniques while training.

Adding these techniques to your self-defense style, you will never regret it because you will know how to defend yourself in any situation, making this martial art style a great advantage. For example, when you find yourself entangled in a street fight, you must be familiar with ways to quickly overshadow and bypass your attacker.

However, when involved in street fights, it takes much more than self-defense to overcome an attack; there must be counter-attacks to form a balance, and Muay Thai does just that for you.

Why Muay Thai Is Important in and Out of the Ring

Self-defense training doesn't only protect you but also others, too. It keeps you physically and emotionally fit and able to defend yourself while increasing your self-esteem and confidence. Learning self-defense helps you stay in shape and healthy; although these techniques demand a lot from you in strength, training, and focus, it has many benefits. The following are more reasons Muay Thai should be considered important for self-defense:

- **Socializing** – It might be an individual sport, but it does open you up to meeting different trainees and trainers during gym sessions and tournaments. Like in the movie "Rocky Balboa," the trainee had a close call with his coach, which gave him an upper hand in the end.
- **Discipline and Focus** – This form of combat requires much dedication and discipline. It requires that you undergo consistent routines and remain focused and determined. If you have yet to master the art of determination, you could easily quit, but Muay Thai naturally helps build discipline.
- **Self-Defense** – In Muay Thai, as you learn the ways of attack, you also know the ways of defense. You must ensure they go hand in hand. Whatever you do, avoid confrontation as a beginner, but if life happens, use your defense skills.
- **Respecting Boundaries** – As much as you want to showcase your skills as you grow, you might be in a situation where you suddenly feel like taking dominance. This is a wrong mindset, and Muay Thai teaches that when you fight, you fight to win, not to kill your opponent. So, it ensures you go easy on those elbows or knockouts.
- **It Builds Confidence** – As discussed earlier, Muay Thai gives you a sense of belonging and strengthens your emotional well-being. You no longer feel easily intimidated, so you walk and talk confidently.

Muay Thai on Ring Defense

In Muay Thai, gaining dominance while in the confines of a ring is an important skill you must have. It doesn't come easy because it takes resilience and skillfulness to get there. Even top fighters lose fights occasionally by miscalculating moves or losing an advantage over their opponents. But in the ring, what increases your confidence is that you know your opponent's weakness and how to override their guard and dominate them.

So, how can you become the best ring fighter? Using a good defense system and moving with speed to counter every attack from your opponent shows you'll dominate the ring. Be ready and in a good stance to counter every attack from an opponent with speed. Make it sharp and unpredictable; this position makes you dominate a ring. When all your moves are sharp and unpredictable, your opponent will fall backward while you're up and pushing.

Using Defense and Counters
- **Catching and Sweeping** – This has many advantages when you use it well as a defender. For example, your opponent throws a kick, and you quickly grab the leg and sweep his other foot off the ground. You could use that measure to strike because, at that point, your opponent has been caught off balance. There are many ways to catch kicks, but it takes precision and timing. With Muay Thai, you cannot be short of ideas for practical ways to catch and sweep your opponent off the ground.
- **Blocking and Counter Attacks** – It is good to defend yourself in a fight, but know that winning a match takes more than blocking and self-defense; you must learn to make counter-attacks when least expected.

Muay Thai on Street Fights

Muay Thai has powerful and lethal techniques, making it even more perfect and interesting for a street fight. Landing a few elbows to your opponent's head or face doesn't take much effort to knock and keep them down. The knees can be lethal, especially when used on your opponent's ribs. Elbows are sharp and land more cuts to the body. The knees are strong and cause more internal injuries.

One main reason Muay Thai is very efficient in street fights is the subtle violence it delivers to the body. The main goal is to strike and stop your attacker from advancing toward you by all means. It's an aggressive and direct move leaving a mark at a strike. It is what makes it different from other sports. You must be good with your kicks, punches, elbows, knees, and trips (to sweep off balance) to have a good defense mechanism in Muay. As you become stronger, you will have a greater chance of defending yourself in a street fight.

So, what are the advantages of using Muay Thai in street fights?

It Permits Close Range Technique

With close combat, there is a conservation of energy and distance between fighters. This practice has been the most popular among martial art practitioners. For example, you can clinch your opponent and throw them off balance during street fights. The clinch is a technique essential in Muay Thai. You get to close the distance between you and your opponent and inflict injuries on them with your knees to their sides or head, giving you more control over the fight – and them.

Street Fights Have Many Grabs

Although it will be considered as a foul if you hold or grab your opponent, unless you want to attack them, you should be alert to their attacks. When you are attacked by an opponent, you should maintain a good stance, and be ready to counter attack at any time. You can do any of these – block the punch, blow or kick, and strike them down. You can also maneuver your opponents by grabbing their attacking limb as a means of self-defense.

A Good Defensive Position

Having your shoulders and feet apart in width gives a good, stable defense stance, giving you easy mobility for a fight. You can have more fluid movements, and your reactions are swift and sharp when you move. Use your elbows to guard your body against attacks and counter-attacks. Another good fighting stance is keeping your hands facing upwards and loose, not tight as in a fist. Hold them up, covering your chin to protect your face from unknown strikes.

Whether you're considering engaging in a ring fight or involved in a street fight, using Muay Thai techniques proves best for self-defense. It is fierce and precise, using eight limbs for combat. To engage in any fight, street, or ring, you must build certain fundamental skills: balance, head movement, tight grip, and guarding your face. You can build your defense using calculated moves with these. For every defense, there must be a counter-attack. So, while gauging your opponent's techniques, strengths, and weaknesses, you should plan to dominate by working on your speed and flexibility. Have a good defensive position and learn to use your elbows for short-distance strikes and your knees to take your opponent off balance.

Chapter 11: Spar Like a Master

Sparring represents one of the most vital components of boxing training. It's the closest thing to a real battle. It helps you better understand how to use the skills and strategies you learned in the gym (regarding range and reach, rhythm and time, and different power levels). This chapter guides you through the sparring basics and ensures you know when best to begin. You will learn sparring etiquette, gear, and other relevant tips, making your beginner sparring journey smooth.

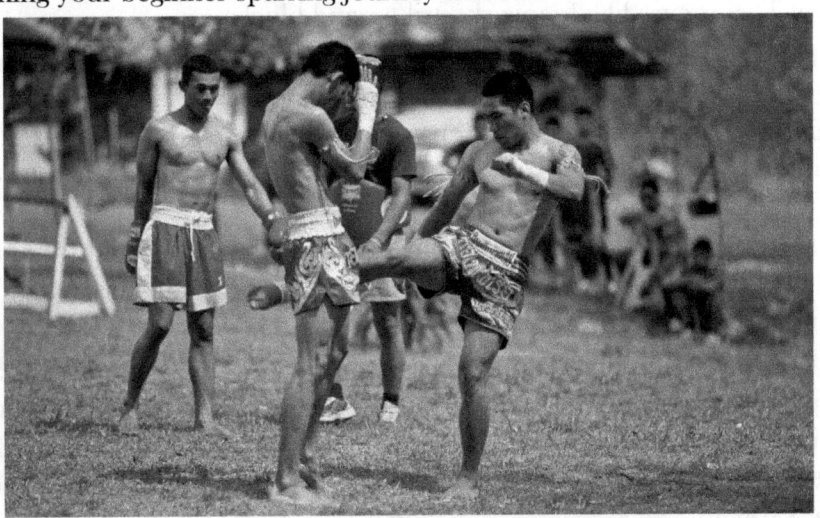

Sparring can help you practice the skills you've learned.
https://commons.wikimedia.org/wiki/File:USMC-120215-M-SR181-138.jpg

Basics of Sparring

Making you and your partner acquainted with the ups and downs of a real battle is the main goal of sparring. It's created to imitate particular events and situations you might encounter in the ring or real life so that you are fully prepared to apply your talents when necessary.

It can be intimidating to spar as a beginner in boxing or kickboxing. The idea of entering the ring and using what you learned against a live subject can make you uneasy. It's a reality you never encountered, and nothing can compare.

However, you will eventually achieve a high level in your training. Your abilities improve, as does your technique. Indeed, sparring is rather intimidating to those uninformed and untrained.

When Does a Beginner Start Sparring?

Many boxers practicing for a few months have frequently pondered when they should begin sparring; this is one of the most commonly asked questions. The response differs from person to person, although sparring should be started after around three to four months of steady, solid training.

It is a good time to begin sparring once you're comfortable with basic Muay Thai moves like footwork, strikes, and blocks.

The fundamentals should be part of your regular workout program. The basic defensive tactical strategies include evading, slipping, countering, and fundamental offensive and defensive combinations. You don't want to rush into a sparring session, so wait until you are sufficiently secure in your skills, at least in theory.

Then, it's time to move on to dueling sessions once you have trained and rehearsed them enough. Your reflexes, timing, and general fighting abilities will then improve.

Asking your coach is another excellent idea to determine if you are prepared to spar. Your coaches can assess your training progress and decide if you have reached the necessary level to test your prowess in the ring against a live opponent. You are certainly ready when your coach thinks you are.

Sparring Gear

The size of your bank account and gym bag is your only restriction when purchasing Muay Thai training equipment. Most beginners can get by with little equipment. Still, after you make a name for yourself, you'll discover that acquiring Muay Thai gear is as fun as engaging in "the practice of eight limbs."

To ensure you are set up correctly, use the following appropriate sparring gear to prevent injuries:

Shin Guards

An important piece of gear for a Muay Thai fighter is the shin guards or shin pads. It protects the shin and foot from strong kicks and blows. They are essential for honing kick-checking reflexes.

Although many sizes and materials are available, the most basic version will work for beginners. Make sure you can move about freely without feeling constrained. Also, ensure they are thick enough to protect you and your companion by offering ample padding.

Ankle Wraps

If you want more support for your ankles, get a pair of ankle wraps. They might not be the first thing you include in your workout bag, but they are equipment your ankles will benefit from.

Sparring Gloves

Your weight index, experience, and fighting style are significant in your selected glove. However, 16-ounce boxing gloves are generally the most preferred option for sparring. You won't strike as hard if you use a 12 or 14-ounce glove because they provide the perfect balance of comfort and protection. Gloves are essential because they safeguard your and your opponent's hands. While gloves are usually available at the gym, getting your own is advisable for acquaintance and personal hygiene.

If you want to try them on, it is best to purchase them in person. The gloves must be properly sized, with adequate wrist support and padding.

Mouth Guard

A quality mouthguard will shield strikes and keep your teeth from breaking or cracking, giving them adequate protection. While you can exert pressure by biting down firmly and keeping your jaw clenched, a mouthguard aids in lowering the risk of concussions or other head injuries. Various mouthguard styles are available, but a boil-and-bite mouthguard is ideal for beginners. Nevertheless, a frequent problem with a boil-and-bite mouthguard is that it occasionally cannot fit properly, hence the reason top athletes wear custom-fitted mouthguards. Although a custom mouthguard is unnecessary for routine training, you could get one for additional safety.

Headgear

Headgear is a smart idea. But don't let it fool you into thinking you're safe. Don't open yourself up to headshots merely because you're wearing headgear. Head traumas do accumulate over time if your gym has a tendency to host intense sparring matches or if you mix Thai boxing with pure boxing. It is sensible to consider donning protective headgear in these circumstances. When selecting the best headgear, you must consider a few things: safety coverage, suitability, visibility, and weight. However, visibility improves with less protection coverage and vice versa.

Like your gloves, the more protection it provides due to denser padding, the heavier the weight, and vice versa. Although a more serious, protective headgear offers superior defense against blows to the head, it can slow down your ability to dodge attacks. The most effective way to prevent head injuries is unquestionably through avoidance. Therefore, the ideal headgear balances sufficient security and high visibility – all within a natural and comfortable fit.

Hand Wraps

Hand wraps shield the 27 small bones in your hands, protecting them (and the soft tissue surrounding them) from harm. Additionally, hand wraps secure your hand so that your fingers and wrists do not move while you punch. Invest in a high-quality pair when purchasing hand wraps because they will serve you longer and provide additional protection. Along with investing in good hand wraps, you must know about proper hand-wrapping techniques.

Groin Guard

Due to the biological and anatomical makeup of men's genitalia (and greater outward positioning), the groin protector is more suitable for men than women. A groin kick is known for shattering many men's sense of self. This soul-crushing torment will leave the strongest men screaming in agony and curled up like a fetus. Keep yourself safe; always wear a groin guard when sparring. It could save your life.

Some practical advice while choosing a groin guard; the family's precious gems should be completely covered by the right groin guard, with no slippage. The guard should be comfy and tightly fitted so that it doesn't move about while you move. Of course, for effective protection against unintentional forceful knocks, the cup must be strong and long-lasting.

Groin guards come in three primary varieties: the jock strap, compression shorts with cups, and Thai steel cups with laces. All have identical goals and different designs. It comes down to personal preference for a good fit and feel when choosing one.

Muay Thai Knee and Elbow Pads

Muay Thai elbow and knee pads are less frequently used during sparring. People with knee injuries or issues or who want more thorough protection typically wear knee pads. Nobody will prevent you from donning knee protectors as an extra measure if you practice Muay Thai for leisure.

The knee pad can minimize the pressure if you strike your sparring partners with knee blows. While elbow strikes are permitted in sparring, elbow pads are worn to lessen damage and safeguard the elbows.

Elbow blows are extremely risky, so most gyms forbid them during sparring. Despite wearing protective gear, elbow blows can be very harmful. As a result, elbow sparring ought to be carried out under professional guidance, and special care must be given when regulating power or pace to prevent bodily harm.

Muay Thai Shorts

Get a pair of Muay Thai shorts because one of the worst things you would want to do is arrive at a Muay Thai gym with basketball shorts. The thighs and groin of Muay Thai shorts are designed with space to strike freely. Perform a couple of kicks while trying on a pair to evaluate if they fit comfortably and provide enough room for kicking.

Comfortable Clothing

Even though most male athletes like to work out only in shorts, ladies must invest in a top that doesn't retain excessive sweat. Veteran martial artists usually advise a sleeveless, form-fitting, and cozy top for women. If you're unsure, get one made expressly for Muay Thai training. Also, procure an ideal pair of workout bras. They have three advantages: they're comfortable, protect your breasts, and are made from ventilated material.

Sparring Etiquette

Below are some sparring etiquettes you must know in Muay Thai:
- Have the required gear
- Keep the contact nice and light; sparring is not a fight
- Always show respect
- Communicate with your sparring partner
- Don't "walk through" punches and kicks

Sparring Tips

The practice of sparring exercises is one of the essential elements for fighters to develop how they fight and gain experience in a real-life combat setting. Muay Thai sparring is intimidating and thrilling for a beginner. Muay Thai sparring assists you in getting ready to apply your abilities correctly when the occasion demands it.

Below are a few sparring beginner tips you should know before you enter the ring with your sparring partner.

Prioritize Your Safety Above All Else

For your first sparring session, the primary and most crucial thing to consider is your safety should always come first. A sparring match must occur in a safe and regulated atmosphere to ensure you and your sparring partner can hone your moves without concern of needless injuries.

Moreover, wearing the correct safety equipment, like headgear, mouthguard, gloves, and protective shin pads, is essential. To increase your training sessions' effectiveness, your coach and other trainers must be on the ground to oversee your sparring sessions.

You Are Not Required to "Win" When Sparring

There is no such thing as "winning" a sparring match. Read that again – and remember it!

There have been numerous sparring sessions, far too often, wherein beginners attempt to kill one another as if it were a title match. This way of thinking causes you to focus excessively on landing powerful blows on your partner while neglecting to hone your technique. Nobody will believe you are a great warrior regardless of whether you did well in one round of sparring.

The trick is to improve. When you spar, you must constantly attempt to do better than what you did previously. Therefore, if this is your first attempt at sparring, you will undoubtedly have a ton of strategies you can practice and perfect. Relax and concentrate mostly on what you can learn from the experience.

Pick an Aspect to Concentrate On

You must decide which areas to improve before your Muay Thai sparring matches. It is crucial since it helps create better-organized training sessions by giving your sparring a specific goal.

Choose a few primary areas to concentrate on throughout your sparring session. For instance, you might use different elbow strikes and combinations in your sparring session if you seek to improve your elbow techniques. Following this process, you polish a particular skill or aspect more effectively.

Ensure Your Coach Approves

Don't be a jerk who enters an unsupervised maiden sparring session. You likely haven't traded blows because your coach thinks you're unprepared. You are not qualified for a sparring match if your coach feels that way.

It is crucial for you and your sparring companions' protection. Many veterans have sparred with folks on their debut sessions, yet they always go crazy, unleashing full-throttle strikes and behaving like it is a brawl. Avoid being *that person*.

Develop a Strategic Plan

Believing that you are playing a game while you spar is useful because, like in any game, developing a winning strategy is essential. The most fundamental principle of Muay Thai is to rack up the most points while preventing your opponent from doing the same. Body kicks get more points in traditional Muay Thai than other techniques like low kicks, knees, and punches. Developing a game plan before your sparring exercise provides a clear path to stick to. Additionally, depending if you operate in defense or attack, you might prefer to select a strategy beforehand.

Have a Wonderful Time

Take things easy and have fun during the process. You should be proud of yourself for having the courage to fight. Always be cordial to your rivals, and enjoy the new bonds you form with your crew of sparring companions.

Muay Thai sparring will help you as a beginner by developing your skills and allowing you to regulate your body.

Chapter 12: Muay Thai vs. Dutch Kickboxing

Now that the basics have been covered, like working on the stance and various offense and defense techniques, let's read about one of the biggest rivalries between two martial art forms. Yes, you read it right. This rivalry is between Muay Thai and Dutch kickboxing – a hot topic for combat sports enthusiasts for several decades.

This chapter compares both fighting styles by listing the key differences between their rules, training, techniques, and relevant information to decide the boxing style that suits you the most.

An Introduction to Dutch Kickboxing

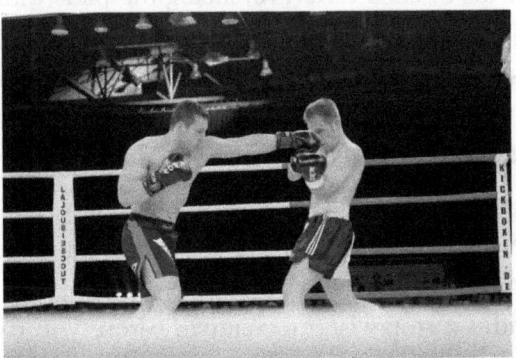

Dutch kickboxing is a combination of Muay Thai and Kyokushin Karate.
Claus Michelfelder, CC BY-SA 4.0 <https://creativecommons.org/licenses/by-sa/4.0>, via Wikimedia Commons: https://commons.wikimedia.org/wiki/File:WKA_World_Championship_2012_Munich_444.JPG

Since the history and origins of Muay Thai have already been covered, let's have a brief overview of this equally popular rival of Muay Thai from the history books.

Dutch Kickboxing is a fusion of Muay Thai, Japanese kickboxing, and Kyokushin karate combat styles and originated in the Netherlands. This fighting style has become popular since it originated and has managed to captivate hundreds and thousands of people to choose Dutch kickboxing. One major difference that sets Dutch kickboxing apart is the Kyokushin karate influence. Dutch kickboxing mostly gets its moves, combos, and techniques from Muay Thai and Japanese kickboxing, but their speed and aggression are from Kyokushin. These boxers always take an aggressive stance to keep the pressure on.

Another general reason differentiating the two combat styles is the heavy use of punches and low kicks for finishing moves.

The Dutch kickboxing style was developed by local karatekas who traveled to Japan to learn Japanese kickboxing and Kyokushin karate. These Dutch boxers returned home to teach these styles, and over time, a mix of these Japanese fighting techniques and Muay Thai gave birth to Dutch kickboxing.

Key Differences

Dutch Kickboxing Training Protocols

The training protocols and drilling techniques in Dutch kickboxing and Muay Thai vary greatly. Dutch kickboxing drills are different in pad work, as there's no need for coaches to hold the pads when drilling. Boxers deliver drills to each other, replacing the pads with boxing gloves.

Dutch sparring is quite popular as training protocols, like without using pads, push the body to its limits, improving results in physical strength and cardiovascular health.

Strengths of Dutch Kickboxing Drills

- Training becomes consistent when you drill with a partner
- Countering moves and using footwork for a better stance are improved
- It provides a step-wise mechanism where you can add new and complex drills as you progress

Drawbacks of Dutch Kickboxing Drills
- Although you can perform drills, there's little to no room for learning new moves or improving existing ones because many fighters are not coaches and can't correct the other person when they make a mistake.
- Using force is limited when striking during drilling because there are no pads to withstand forceful impacts.
- You repeat the same drills as opposed to drilling under the supervision of a coach.
- You won't receive instant feedback from the coach or know the correct moves to make.

Muay Thai Training Protocols

Using forearm and belly pads is required during Muay Thai training. During Muay Thai drilling, most fighters have an experienced partner or a coach holding the pads. These training partners also wear shin and instep protectors to throw kicks during drilling to improve reflexes further.

One significant difference to mention in Muay Thai and Dutch kickboxing training is related to a technique known as clinching. You'll only see clinching and its training in a Muay Thai gym because all other combat sports have restricted or excluded this technique.

Strengths of Muay Thai Drilling
- You get massive chances of improving your techniques and combos as the coach will be there to correct your techniques.
- Since coaches are trained to improve the fighter's skills, it gives the fighter a window of opportunity to experiment with different tempos, rhythms, and ranges to polish their skills.
- You won't worry about the impact and can unleash your full power when training.
- The training session won't be limited to punches only. You can try every technique with ease.

Drawbacks of Muay Thai Training
- Not every pad holder can take the impact of strikes when training. If the pad holder is not doing their job effectively, it lowers the fighter's chances of polishing their skills.

- Poor pad handling can make the fighter develop ineffective or wrong techniques.

While drilling in Dutch kickboxing is all about repeating combinations or drilling for a specific set of rounds, Muay Thai maintains a more laidback approach with no specific drilling sets or repeating the same exercises. Furthermore, under the supervision of a coach, developing new skills and refining existing skills becomes much easier.

Pad Usage

Using pads for training pad work is mostly seen in Muay Thai than in Dutch Kickboxing, mainly because most Dutch kickboxing gyms avoid incorporating them during training sessions. However, it doesn't mean these pads are banned or cannot be used; it's merely a matter of preference. In contrast, many gyms and Dutch Kickboxing coaches regularly use these training pads while training their fighters.

Before moving further, addressing another misconception is necessary. Many people believe you only use punches and low kicks in Dutch kickboxing. However, that's only partially true. You can use your knees and elbows and throw a few high kicks like Muay Thai. If you're still confused and might think that if all the moves are in both fighting styles, then what makes them different?

The answer is the fighter's attitude or stance in both combat styles. For example, a Muay Thai fighter will throw a bunch of moves and use techniques strategically to weaken their opponent. In contrast, a Dutch kickboxer always maintains an aggressive stance and focuses on the volume of strikes. The most volume can only be delivered through punches -the main difference between these robust combat sports forms.

The Differences in Techniques

This section compares techniques to know their differences and better understand the reasons that set these two combat styles apart.

Punching

Using punches is similar to Western boxing, but Dutch kickboxing has a few added variations, like the Superman punch or the back fist. Instead of working on a variety of punches, Dutch kickboxing is more about maintaining an aggressive stance and delivering impactful strikes while moving forward.

On the other hand, Muay Thai fighters use a different approach to using punches. Rather than delivering a high volume of punches at a fast pace, Muay Thai fighters use a combination of techniques for effective results. For example, they might throw a left jab and immediately clinch the opponent to pin them to the ground or use a mix of knee strikes and punches to create an opening for the next strike.

In a nutshell, a Dutch kickboxer will focus on their pace and the volume of attacks, but a Muay Thai fighter will always incorporate different techniques together and execute them strategically for the desired outcomes.

Kicking

If you are not a boxer, it might be difficult to understand the differences in the kicking style. While you will find identical techniques in both fighting styles, the way and the frequency with which they are executed varies. For example, in a Dutch kickboxing match, the emphasis is on delivering a high volume of punches and low kicks. However, Muay Thai has more room for different kicking techniques instead of relying on only a few.

Knee Strikes

Using knee swings and targeting the legs with knees can only be seen in Muay Thai. However, using knee strikes to the face is common in Dutch kickboxing. When executed properly, this lethal strike can knock out the opponent within a few seconds.

(Likewise, Muay Thai boxers use lethal elbow strikes to knock out opponents.)

Stance

The stance Dutch kickboxers take is more squared and dynamic. They always place their feet close, so their stance allows heavy striking and quick movements. Without maintaining a firm stance, they cannot use their upper body effectively and throw punches to potentially knock out the enemy. When making a guarding stance, the head and face are the main areas a Dutch kickboxer is focused on to protect.

In contrast, Muay Thai boxers focus on a stance for being prepared for action, but in a slightly relaxed manner. Their feet are placed wider and are angled, making it easier to use kicking techniques, maintain balance, and improve mobility. The guarding position in Muay Thai is focused on protecting the midsection and lower body instead of only the face. This guarding position in Muay Thai enables boxers to counter incoming strikes using various counter techniques and to minimize the impact these strikes have on the body.

Striking Techniques

When striking in Dutch kickboxing, the main emphasis is throwing powerful punches and adding low kicks. This combination is quite popular and is even elevated by some enthusiasts to an art form. The delivered strikes are lightning-fast and transition from punches to low kicks and back again in the blink of an eye. The punches are aimed at the face or an opening on the upper body, and low kicks are aimed at the legs.

On the contrary, Muay Thai incorporates a massive combination of moves stemming from the art of eight limbs. The mix of jabs, kicks, elbow strikes, and grapples can break the opponent's spirits and turn the tides. Whether the opponent is in short or long range, there are moves and endless offensive and defensive combinations to use against the opponent.

Clinching

Clinching in Muay Thai makes it different from Dutch kickboxing, as many Muay Thai fighters mix clinching with elbow, knee, and forearm strikes to target different body areas. Unlike Muay Thai, Dutch kickboxing clinching is only done occasionally, like when the opponent is too near for an attempt to look for openings to strike. Clinching is also done to land a few strikes and create distance.

As mentioned, clinching is one of the core techniques used in Muay Thai and more than in other combat sports. These fighters put endless hours into training and perfecting the techniques to win fights. In Muay Thai, boxers are always on the lookout for an opening to initiate a grapple, use several clinching techniques, and find opportunities to land strikes that can make their opponent lose their balance or other techniques like sweeps and knee strikes.

Fighting Style

Dutch kickboxing's fighting style is kept aggressive by throwing a series of powerful punches and low kicks. This approach maintains pressure on the opponent. With each strike, a Dutch kickboxer moves forward to overpower the opponent and control the duel's pace, rhythm, and tempo.

On the other side of the picture, Muay Thai boxers are trained to endure impactful strikes and blows, sustain damage, and constantly seek the opponent's weaknesses. Maintaining this attitude and deciphering the weak points allows these boxers to plan their next move effectively. Effective countermoves and hitting hard at the right time make a Muay Thai fighter different than their rival combat sport, Dutch kickboxing.

Training Emphasis

Although we have already explained some differences in training, let's take a deeper dive. The training in Dutch kickboxing focuses on developing strength and stamina to primarily maintain an aggressive stance and deliver one powerful strike after another to assert dominance in the game. Their drills are high-intensity and aimed at improving physical strength and agility.

While Dutch kickboxers work on a specific skill set, Muay Thai boxers maintain a holistic approach striving to balance techniques, strength, agility, and fluidity. Furthermore, Muay Thai boxers spend most of their training session improving their clinching techniques. Their approach is well-rounded, and they are always ready to face varying situations in the ring.

Fighting Distance

Dutch kickboxing favors a medium to long-range fighting distance between opponents. In contrast, Muay Thai can fight at long, medium, and close ranges without issue. Close combat in Muay Thai can result in a knockout as the boxer can land their clinching moves and throw knee strikes for a knockout. A Dutch kickboxer might not be comfortable switching the fighting distance like a Muay Thai boxer who can change their stance and execute a new set of moves in the blink of an eye.

Defensive Techniques

The counter moves a Dutch kickboxer aims to evade the strikes and minimize their impact. While defending, the boxer promptly changes their foot placement and posture and simultaneously throws offensive strikes whenever a window of opportunity opens.

Like the offensive moves, Muay Thai has a massive range of defensive techniques and combinations to counter virtually every incoming strike. Blocking the attacks, parries, and redirecting the attack are common defensive techniques. Clinching is also a defensive tool effectively used to limit the number of attacks and reduce their impact.

Fighting Culture

Although both combat sports forms have several differences, a clear difference is their fighting culture. While Dutch kickboxing is a hybrid combat style mainly influenced by other professional martial arts and combat sport forms and is competitive, Muay Thai has deep roots in the region's culture and traditions. A Dutch kickboxer will maintain a professional, organized, and structured approach in training. In contrast, pre-fight dances, post-fight ceremonial events, and paying homage to their ancestors and teachers are expressions Muay Thai fighters exhibit the most.

Scoring System

Some evident differences are in the scoring systems. In a Dutch kickboxing match, landing clean strikes on target areas will score points. Similarly, knocking out the opponent impacts the final score. While Muay Thai awards a similar score for knockouts and clean strikes, an additional emphasis is put on the strikes made during clinching. Defending effectively and asserting dominance throughout the game are other factors affecting the final score.

Finalizing Your Pick

Before choosing any combat style, it's crucial to understand the following factors to decide the fighting style that suits you best.

Training Environment

The environment in which you train will define the learning outcomes. Working out in a training environment resonating with your inner self provides a sense of relaxation, and acting as a sanctuary will make you step up your game to the next level. Regardless of the combat sport you select, the gym or training institute you enroll in must have a supportive community, a learning atmosphere, and coaches with enough experience to unlock your true potential. Along the way, you'll forge unbreakable relationships with other members and share the same passion to push you forward whenever you feel low.

Personal Goals

Take time off and dwell in your inner self to understand your preference. For example, if you are spiritual and ready to embark on a cultural journey connecting deeply to your training, then Muay Thai would be a feasible choice. On the contrary, Dutch kickboxing might be the answer if you want to maintain a more professional training-based approach and develop self-confidence. Nevertheless, exploring your personal goals and preferences will guide you to the combat style aligning best with your aspirations.

Fighting Style

Picture both combat styles in your mind and evaluate whether you will be comfortable with close-range combat, clinching, and delivering impactful strikes. Or would you like to take the pressure up a notch and prefer delivering constant strikes to the opponent? Choose the fighting style that resonates with you the most so it becomes easier to train, learn, and master these combat styles.

Physical Demands

Although both are physically demanding sports activities, being physically fit is crucial if you want to opt for training. Furthermore, the physical demands of both styles vary slightly. For example, Muay Thai requires a balance of strength and endurance. In contrast, Dutch kickboxing focuses more on being agile to deliver consistent strikes. Watching a few matches of both fighting styles will make it easier to decide.

In a nutshell, the choice between Muay Thai and Dutch kickboxing should always be influenced by a person's preferences and goals. If you want to experience the cultural connection and are fine with balancing striking, clinching, defense, and strength activities, Muay Thai is an excellent choice. However, Dutch kickboxing is the perfect sport if you are fast-paced and want to keep asserting your dominance over the opponent while constantly landing strikes.

Taking Trial Sessions

The best way you can learn a combat sport is through hands-on experience. Several gyms and clubs offer trial sessions which are mostly free or have a nominal fee. Whichever martial arts discipline you choose, you'll face challenges while training, but it will benefit improving your basic fighting skills.

Attending a few trial classes, you will grasp the basic movements, techniques, and related moves to better judge if you are physically and mentally capable of training and competing in combat sports. Since most gyms want new members to join, they occasionally offer fee waivers and discounts, saving you much more money than purchasing a membership for regular days.

Cost of the Program

Most gyms and combat sports clubs have paid membership plans of varying amounts and services. Evaluating every cost related to your training should be calculated beforehand. For example, consider the training fee, the cost of the gear, and other related fees so you know how much money to put aside for these training sessions.

It's always tempting to pick a gym or a training class that costs the least, but you won't get your value for money in most situations. It's better to commit to a gym by evaluating their services and knowing you will learn the combat sport to compete or just to indulge in a physically fun activity while learning self-defense. Finding the answers to these questions will make your choice more solid, suiting you best.

Nonetheless, never compromise on the quality of training and the instructor's experience in the relevant combat sport. The better the training quality and coaching, the better the results in learning the martial arts form. Therefore, having a reputable training environment with the required facilities is imperative if you want to improve your game.

Chapter 13: Daily Training Drills

Are you looking to sharpen your daily routine? Or do you want to mix up your fitness regime? Whatever your daily fitness regimen goals, this comprehensive chapter has what it takes.

In this last chapter, you will discover many ways to build a daily Muay Thai workout plan catered specifically toward beginners (within the confines of your dwelling place or a local fitness center). From tried and tested routines to proven effective training techniques, expect nothing less from this packed chapter.

Working on Your Stretching, Mobility, and Hip Rotation

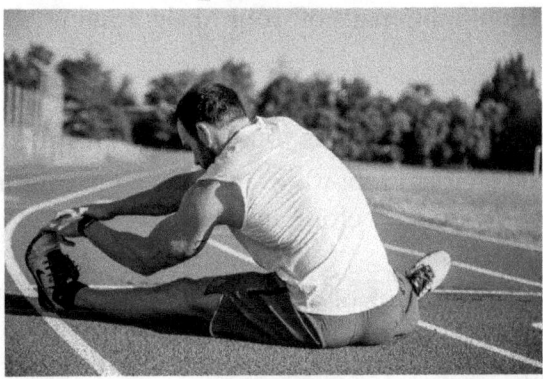

Stretching, flexibility, and mobility are necessary for Muay Thai.
https://unsplash.com/photos/WX7FSaiYxK8?utm_source=unsplash&utm_medium=referral&utm_content=creditShareLink

When most people reflect on their first day of Muay Thai training, they realize that focusing on hip rotation, flexibility, posture, and mobility would have made them better fighters. Properly executing hip rotation is essential since it determines how much power you can put into your kicks and knee strikes. Surprisingly, anyone can practice these exercises with minimal resources anywhere.

Good Hip Rotation

Consider if someone broke into your home: would you swing a baseball bat vertically or use your hips to generate full force? In Muay Thai, kicking correctly depends on proper hip rotation. An inexperienced fighter attempting upward motion kicks could lead to unintended effects like self-injury instead of effectively striking the intended opponent.

Similarly, when executing a roundhouse kick in Muay Thai, always keep the following in mind:

- Extend your lead leg's heel beyond your toes while rotating it 180 degrees in line with the kick direction
- To execute a more effective kick, focus on directing your force upward instead of downward
- Additionally, swiftly swing your arm, using the same one as your kicking leg, while propelling your shoulder forward

The key to accurately performing this technique is activating your lateral gluteal muscles while rotating your hip; you will feel a specific sensation telling you when you've got it right. While unconventional in Muay Thai, mastering proper hip rotation is crucial for efficient kicks. This exercise should be part of your daily routine to enhance hip flexibility.

1. Start by placing one foot on an elevated surface like a sofa and the other foot on tiptoes as you would do preparing to kick.
2. Rotate the elevated foot while engaging your arms and repeat this sequence 25 times before switching legs and repeating it 100 times on each leg.
3. Aim for a minimum of 100 repetitions daily on both legs and even up to 300 reps per leg if you have tight hips, as they do in Thailand.

Mobility

If you live a sedentary lifestyle in the Western world, your hips are likely tight. This impacts your athletic performance when executing kicks, particularly in sports like Muay Thai boxing.

Luckily, there are ways you can regain hip mobility independently. Maintaining proper hip rotation is essential for professional athletes and minimizing injuries during physical activities like soccer games.

Research on injury prevention among professional athletes who incorporated muscle-mobility exercises into their training regime has shown impressive outcomes. Practicing alone provides an excellent opportunity to improve movement quality patterns.

One excellent video clip shared by Don Heatrick provided beneficial advice aimed at assisting Muay Thai practitioners in unlocking their hip joints. The routines highlighted therein have proven remarkably successful in enhancing kicking techniques, regardless of form.

You can significantly improve your hip flexibility by following the instructions outlined in this section and carrying out all three daily exercise routines using materials like foam rollers, lacrosse balls, and resistant bands (available at affordable prices on Amazon).

1. Releasing Your Hips
- To start, place a foam roller just above your knees before gradually moving it up along your thighs, which aids in breaking down muscle tissue more effectively.
- If tight spots arise while doing this exercise, gently move your leg from left to right, targeting troubled tissues while flexing the hip joint muscles.
- Ignore IT (iliotibial) bands located midway since they are prone to injury if rolled on directly.

2. Opening Your Hips
1. Secure one end of a resistance band tightly onto solid structures like squat racks or TV stands.
2. Step into the band with it placed high behind the gluteal muscles so there's significant tension pulling at your hips.
3. Initiate the movement by squeezing the glutes tightly and tilting the pelvis forward, propelling the hip joint in front of the knee.

4. Do not over-arch your back while prioritizing mobility at the hips. Specifically, switching up stances helps you practice from different angles.
5. Set aside 1-2 minutes for continuous repetitions on each side before moving on.

3. Anchoring Your Hips

Stabilizing the hips takes more than just following any old workout routine; it takes effort, precision, and technique.

- The best way to get started is to find a solid platform, a bench, or a chair that matches up perfectly with where your foot needs support.
- Once you've located this footing, ensure when positioning yourself on it, one hip sits lower than or lines up exactly at knee level; this ensures proper alignment throughout the execution.
- Furthermore, keep good posture during every step: chest upright and chin pointing downward.
- By exerting force from underfoot while simultaneously engaging the glute muscles (feel free to savor the gentle stretch), you'll be effectively stabilizing your hips in no time.
- Lastly, incorporate weights into the mix and aim for three sets of ten reps per leg to test your limits.

Do you want to take your Muay Thai performance to another level? Then do these exercises; they'll enhance your overall well-being and have powerful effects on muscle length, joint alignment, neuromuscular control, and pivotal components in optimizing range of motion for improved fighting ability.

Ensure you integrate these exercises into a robust warm-up routine with dynamic moves to ensure correct kick execution while decreasing the risk of harm from bad movement patterns.

The release and opening of the hips can happen any time during the day as an active rest technique between weightlifting sessions or partake in designated recovery days while addressing postural issues and decreasing muscle discomfort.

Investing in high-quality gear is paramount to attaining the maximum benefits of these Muay Thai exercises and maintaining good posture.

However, today's technological advancements like smartphones and computers have led to poor posture, resulting in future health complications. But fret not. The various routines outlined above aid in releasing tension from the hips and stabilizing them.

Stretching

In Muay Thai, where precision matters greatly, taking time out for stretching greatly enhances your overall performance. Once you have warmed up appropriately with mobility exercises, focus on lengthening your muscles through stretching.

Regular stretching results in better flexibility, translating into improved agility when performing strikes or kicks that need maneuverability from your body. Moreover, going through an extensive stretch regime before training or competitions aids in injury prevention by creating greater elasticity in muscles.

1. Warm Up

Don't skip warming up before starting any stretching exercises because you don't want to risk muscle strains or pulls. Begin with some easy aerobic activities like jogging or jumping jacks for 5-10 minutes to get your blood flowing and muscles prepped for stretching.

2. Dynamic Stretches

Dynamic stretches are great as warm-ups and as movements simulating what you do during training or competitions. They improve blood circulation, expand the range of motion, and condition the muscles. Dynamic stretches include leg swings, arm circles, and torso twists. To carry out dynamic stretches, do the following:

1. Stand next to a wall or other stable structure and swing one leg back and forth while keeping balance; repeat 10-15 times per leg.
2. Continue with arms extended sideways from your shoulder, making small clockwise circular motions, gradually increasing size until you feel stretched enough.
3. Keep things fresh by alternating the direction of your twists; switch to counterclockwise after a few rotations.
4. Stand with feet shoulder-width apart and place your hands on the hips before making torso twists – rotating the upper body from left to right and back again.

3. Static Stretches

Static stretches are a good option targeting several key muscle groups to improve flexibility during stretching sessions. These exercises require you to hold positions for roughly 15-30 seconds, which helps loosen tightness in those areas.

After completing warm-ups or exercises, do your best to focus on performing proper techniques and holding positions as long as possible. A static stretch should focus on muscle groups like the hamstring, quadriceps, chest, shoulder, hip flexor, triceps, and groin.

- The hamstring stretch is one method that entails sitting down on a flat surface with one leg extended straight while bending the other before leaning forward slightly, reaching toward the toes with your back straight.
- Quadriceps stretching is another beneficial technique for improving flexibility by pulling corresponding heels (opposite side) toward the buttocks without curving your back while remaining balanced and standing tall.
- When targeting the chest muscles, use doorways by placing the forearm against the frame before leaning forward gently for an effective stretch.
- Incorporating shoulder and hip flexor stretching could be beneficial. Extend your arms across your body or kneel with one knee on flat ground while extending the opposite leg ahead for better results.
- Are you seeking to ease pent-up tension in those hip flexor muscles? Simply maintain a proper standing posture and thrust forward from the hips for a couple of rounds, each time swapping back and forth between the left and right side until you detect pleasant stretching sensations.
- For your triceps region, raise one arm high above your head, and bring it back toward the scruff of your neck before slightly tugging at the elbow with the opposite hand for added intensity until you sense beneficial pulling sensations. Repeat this procedure on the other arm.
- You can also address the groin area by sitting down with feet touching each other and the knees extending outwards. While keeping a firm grasp on both feet with your hands, pull inward

using elbows against knees to maximize stretch across this region.

4. Proprioceptive Neuromuscular Facilitation

If you're searching for more challenging stretching techniques requiring interaction, give PNF (proprioceptive neuromuscular facilitation) stretching a try. This unique approach combines strategic muscle contractions with relaxation periods to increase flexibility and expand the range of motion in various body parts.

To get started, try this uncomplicated PNF stretch focusing on the hamstrings:

1. Begin by laying on your back with one leg lifted in the air
2. Position yourself so that you can easily reach your ankle with one hand while extending the arm outwards to meet your partner's grasp with their other hand.
3. Now engage in an intense push-pull routine where you push against their grip toward them, using every bit of effort for 6-10 seconds before finally relaxing.
4. Your partner will continue guiding your leg forward and gently pushing it into greater extension at each progressive round lasting 20-30 seconds.
5. Test each leg until both are equally stretched out.

5. Foam Rolling Stretching

Foam rolling is an effective method to relieve muscle tension and enhance flexibility in different parts of the body through self-myofascial release. For this technique to work wonders on tightness issues, you need a foam roller to target the specific muscles requiring attention.

- To alleviate tightness in quadriceps muscles along the front upper part of the thighs, lie face down with a foam roller under the thighs. Maneuver the roller from your hip area to just above the kneecaps; stop at tender points along this path.
- Similarly, targeting the hamstrings requires seating upright using a foam roller under both thighs. Glide it smoothly upward from your glutes toward your knees, putting even pressure on sore areas encountered during this process.
- If the calf muscles are causing trouble, sit on the ground with the legs straight, using slow rolling movements to slowly work

upward along each section.
- Relief of upper-back pains can be achieved by lying flat on your back and placing a cylindrical foam roller under your shoulder blades. Move the foam roller up and down your spine gently.
- Ensure to stop and stay still whenever you come across tender areas.

Daily Shadowboxing Regimen

Every Muay Thai training routine requires a strong foundation for exceptional performance, something shadowboxing can deliver thanks to its multiple advantages, like refining techniques, intricate footwork patterns, and enhancing distance control capabilities.

Below are some priceless tips to derive maximum gain from daily shadowboxing drills:

- Always begin by warming up sufficiently before diving into practice sessions, a routine aimed at preparing muscles appropriately for upcoming intense workouts.
- Utilize dynamic stretching alongside joint rotations, finishing with light cardio exercises like skipping rope or jumping jacks. This activates the muscles early and reduces the likelihood of muscle sprains or strains during subsequent workouts.
- You should choose a spacious area allowing unrestricted mobility without the risk of hazardous elements or barriers. With ample room, you can confidently perform defensive techniques and execute a wide range of striking moves with maximum precision and impact.
- To maximize the effectiveness of shadowboxing during training, it is advisable to mentally visualize an opponent standing in front of you before starting each session. Visualize their movements, anticipate their strikes, and imagine yourself immersed in intense combat scenarios for a more focused approach.
- Perfect your stance and guard position by assuming a balanced position allowing easy transition between offensive and defensive modes. Always keep your feet shoulder-width apart with the lead foot slightly turned outward.
- Ensure you have a raised guard posture covering the face; tuck your chin down while keeping both elbows close to the body

sides for added protection.
- During shadow boxing sessions, incorporate various striking techniques starting from basic moves like jabs, crosses, hooks, and uppercuts using proper techniques before advancing slowly to more difficult ones like elbows, knees, or kicks.
- Always maintain fluid motion without sacrificing precision and power.
- To improve your Muay Thai boxing defense tactics, refine your ability to block or evade incoming strikes by incorporating methods like slipping, ducking, weaving, or parrying while keeping a sturdy guard position on the move. With the power of visualization, imagine going up against different opponents' attacking styles while practicing swift ways of dodging them with quick reflexes through repetition.
- Timing is crucial in accurately landing power hits during fights. Hence, it would be wise to regularly include shadowboxing techniques in training routines to visualize your rival's movements before delivering well-timed counter-strikes

Cardio

This section outlines key exercises and techniques below to help you incorporate cardio into daily Muay Thai training:
- Before starting a workout program, determine what you want from adding more cardio to boost endurance or improve cardiovascular fitness.
- Warming up is necessary to prepare properly before an intense cardio session. Engage in dynamic stretching movements like arm circles, torso twists, or leg swings, which loosen up muscles, boost blood flow, lower the risk of injury, and increase performance levels.
- Ensure correct form throughout to enhance performance in future matches. Engaging in kick and punch pad workouts with a training buddy or coach can greatly improve your cardio endurance while refining your striking techniques. Using the pads, you encounter resistance mimicking the intensity of a genuine fight, urging you to exert maximum effort.
- Running has always been popular for boosting cardiovascular fitness. It enhances leg muscle strength and improves stamina

and endurance levels remarkably.
- Consider incorporating steady-state runs, hill sprints, or interval runs into your regimen to add variety to running sessions.
- Circuit training might be a perfect choice for an all-encompassing full-body workout that blends strength exercises with cardio intervals (like push-ups, squats, burpees, and kettlebell swings). Progress through each exercise promptly without breaks in between for maximum benefit.
- Bag work sessions at high intensity are another excellent addition to your training program. They encourage explosive strikes while combining techniques and swift movements and improving cardio-respiratory endurance by challenging you to maintain a rapid pace throughout each round.
- Whether recovering from intense workouts or just wanting to rest your joints from high-impact activities, swimming laps, or engaging in water-based interval training can help enhance cardiovascular function while protecting vulnerable areas.

This last chapter provided multiple alternatives for establishing an effective daily Muay Thai training program suitable for every environment. Committing yourself to these exercises over time will enable advancement and proficiency in techniques and physical endurance. Last, please do not neglect the utmost importance of safety; always be vigilant and seek expert advice if in doubt. Remember, enjoy yourself in every aspect of mastering this incredible martial art.

Conclusion

Thailand's kickboxing has a centuries-long history and is now an art accepted worldwide. This combat form requires using your eight limbs, and as a beginner, you will make striking moves with kicks, elbows, punches, and your knees.

These are weapons a Muay Thai fighter uses, making it stand out from other combat sports. Centuries ago, Muay Thai fights were often brutal; today, it has been modified, making it a safer competitive sport with referees recording scores and prioritizing safety.

Although Muay Thai is a modern-age sport, it doesn't make it safe for everyone. Still, you can learn the foundations of this combat sport and become a professional fighter with proper learning and coaching. The combat sport might seem dangerous to a beginner who views it through an outdoor lens, but with Muay Thai, there are better ways to learn the techniques, making it as friendly as other sports.

One great benefit of Muay Thai is it brings out an inner warrior within you. It keeps you physically and emotionally fit while exposing you to real-life attack scenarios during training. It is an excellent way to learn self-defense and teaches you how to remain calm when faced with real-life opponents. With Muay Thai, you can confidently enter the ring or fight. While you train, you build stamina and stance, enhancing your concentration skills.

Now that you've been exposed to these practical tips and techniques on Muay Thai, you should put everything into practice. This guide is written so that it leads you through every technique simply and understandably. So, take those steps, hit the gym, train under a coach, set a routine, and ensure you're accountable to someone.

You might burn out in the first few months of training, but that's fine; it's part of the process. Don't give up. While you train, you must practice each technique you learn with other trainees; start cautiously and use protective equipment for sensitive areas.

Muay Thai is one of the most practical and fierce martial art forms. Good luck on your journey to mastering it!

Here's another book by Clint Sharp that you might like

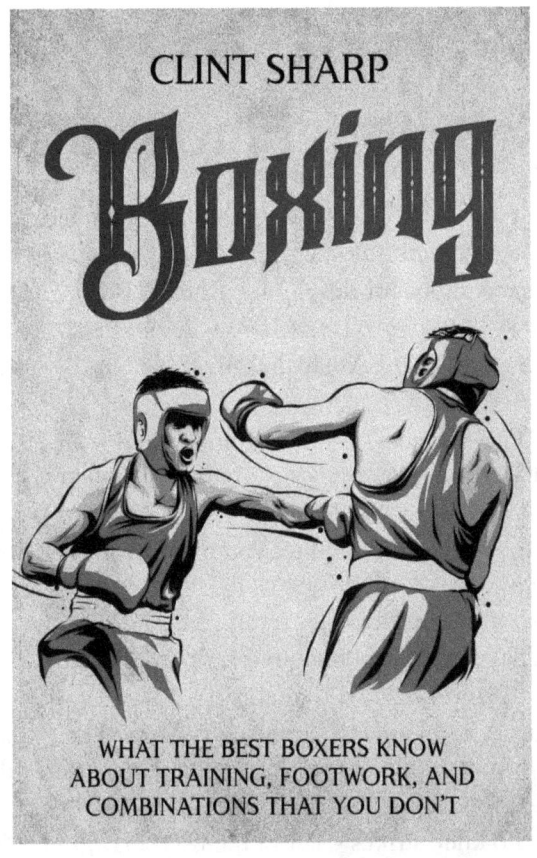

References

10 types of muay Thai kicks. (2019, December 11). Fijimuaythai.com. https://fijimuaythai.com/types-of-muay-thai-kicks/

14 FAV Muay Thai combos for developing RHYTHM & FLOW. (n.d.). Mmashredded.com. https://www.mmashredded.com/blog/muay-thai-combos

5 essential clinching tips. (n.d.). Muay-thai-guy.com. https://www.muay-thai-guy.com/blog/5-essential-clinching-tips

5 essential Muay Thai sparring tips for beginners. (n.d.). 5 Essential Muay Thai Sparring Tips for Beginners. https://www.ubudmuaythai.com/blog/5-essential-muay-thai-sparring-tips-for-beginners

5 essential Muay Thai sweep techniques you must know – evolve university blog. (2023, March 2). Evolve University. https://evolve-university.com/blog/5-essential-muay-thai-sweep-techniques-you-must-know/

A typical Muay Thai workout routine. (n.d.). Muay-Thai-guy.com. https://www.muay-thai-guy.com/blog/muay-thai-workout

Alexis. (2022, August 28). Dutch Kickboxing vs Muay Thai: what are the differences? Mejiro Gym Bali. https://mejirogymbali.com/blog/dutch-kickboxing-vs-muay-thai-differences/

Beginner's GuideTo knee strikes – law of the fist. (2019, June 22). Lawofthefist.com. https://lawofthefist.com/a-beginners-intro-to-the-art-of-knee-strikes/

Best Muay Thai sparring gear. (2019, April 14). Muay Thai Citizen; Kay. https://www.muaythaicitizen.com/best-muay-thai-sparring-gear/

Bryan, A. (2023, January 5). Muay Thai & spirituality. Black Belt Magazine. https://blackbeltmag.com/muay-thai-spirituality

Bryan, A. (n.d.). The ultimate guide to the Muay Thai clinch. Muay-thai-guy.com. https://www.muay-thai-guy.com/blog/clinching-for-muay-thai

Delp, C. (2004). Muay Thai: Traditionen – Grundlagen – Techniken des Thaiboxens (1st ed.). Motorbuch.

Dillon. (2020, May 27). How to practice Muay Thai by yourself: My daily routine. Oneshotmma. https://oneshotmma.com/how-to-practice-muay-thai-by-yourself-my-weekly-routine/

Dunk. (2017, February 15). Common Muay Thai routines when training in Thailand: Part I. Muay Thai; Bokun Wordpress Theme. https://kstmuaythai.com/common-muay-thai-routines-when-training-in-thailand-part-1/

Evolve Vacation. (2018, November 20). How to develop powerful knees in Muay Thai. Evolve Vacation. https://evolve-vacation.com/blog/how-to-develop-powerful-knees-in-muay-thai/

Evolve, M. M. A. (2016, March 23). 7 Muay Thai principles that will make you A better fighter. Evolve Daily. https://evolve-mma.com/blog/7-muay-thai-principles-that-will-make-you-a-better-fighter/

Evolve, M. M. A. (2018, January 15). Muay Thai 101: The roundhouse kick. Evolve Daily. https://evolve-mma.com/blog/muay-thai-101-the-roundhouse-kick/

Evolve, M. M. A. (2020, September 9). The beginner's guide to boxing sparring: 10 things to know. Evolve Daily. https://evolve-mma.com/blog/the-beginners-guide-to-boxing-sparring-10-things-to-know/

Evolve, M. M. A. (2022, February 10). The complete Muay Thai Beginner's Guide. Evolve Daily. https://evolve-mma.com/blog/the-complete-muay-thai-beginners-guide/

Evolve, M. M. A. (2022, June 21). Here's how to utilize sweeps for Muay Thai. Evolve Daily. https://evolve-mma.com/blog/heres-how-to-utilize-sweeps-for-muay-thai/

Evolve, M. M. A. (2022, October 24). Comparing Muay Thai to Dutch kickboxing. Evolve Daily. https://evolve-mma.com/blog/comparing-muay-thai-to-dutch-kickboxing/

Explorer, K. L. (2015, November 24). Muay Thai. Https://www.khaolakexplorer.com/; Khao Lak Explorer. https://www.khaolakexplorer.com/muay-thai/

Hughes, L. (2023, January 26). The Muay Thai workout routine that will get you into shape. Prime Women | An Online Magazine; Prime Women | Online Lifestyle Media for Women over 50. https://primewomen.com/wellness/fitness/muay-thai-workout-routine/

James, K. (2017, January 13). The 8 punches of muay Thai. Fightrr.com. https://fightrr.com/muay-thai/technique/punches

Jones, A. (2023, April 2). Dutch Kickboxing vs. Muay Thai. Fight Falcon – Fight With Style. https://fightfalcon.com/dutch-kickboxing-vs-muay-thai/

Mohan, C. (2020, March 5). Muay Thai training gear you must have in your gym bag. ONE Championship - The Home Of Martial Arts. https://www.onefc.com/lifestyle/muay-thai-training-gear-you-must-have-in-your-gym-bag/

Muay Sok: The Elbow Fighter (June 8th, 2022), Jacob Garner. Muay Sok https://muaythai.com/muay-sok/

Muay Thai – philosophy, techniques, training tips, and more. (n.d.). Ninjaphd.com. https://www.ninjaphd.com/muay-thai/

Muay Thai Guy (2023), 10 Key Muay Thai Defense Techniques Every Fighter Must Know. https://www.muay-thai-guy.com/blog/muay-thai-defense-techniques

Muay Thai history. (2016, March 4). World Thai Boxing Association. https://thaiboxing.com/about/muay-thai-history/

Muay Thai sparring 2023: 10 tips for beginners & more. (2023, March 12). Way of the Fighter. https://wayofthefighter.com/muay-thai-sparring/

Muay Thai Techniques. (n.d.). Blogspot.com. http://muay-thai-techniquess.blogspot.com/2011/06/muay-thai-techniques-clinch-and-neck.html

MuayThaiCitizen, (May 19th, 2022), Kay, Is Muay Thai effective in a Street Fight? https://www.muaythaicitizen.com/is-muay-thai-effective-in-a-street-fight/#:~:text=So%20is%20Muay%20Thai%20effective,of%20controlling%20what%20happens%20next

OneFc (June 30th, 2020), John Wolcott, The 5 Fundamentals Of A Solid Muay Thai Defense. https://www.onefc.com/lifestyle/the-5-fundamentals-of-a-solid-muay-thai-defense/,

Shutts, I. (2018, October 14). Muay Thai boxing and punches. LowKick MMA. https://www.lowkickmma.com/muay-thai-boxing-and-punches

Singpatong-sitnumnoi (December 4th, 2012), Elbow Techniques In Muay Thai http://www.singpatong-sitnumnoi.com/elbow-techniques-in-muay-thai/,

Thailand, M. (2021, February 16). Muay Thai knees. Muay Thailand. https://www.muaythailand.co.uk/blogs/techniques/muay-thai-knees

The 10 best beginner Muay Thai sparring tips. (n.d.). Muay-thai-guy.com. https://www.muay-thai-guy.com/blog/beginner-muay-thai-sparring-tips

The ultimate guide to Muay Thai knees – evolve university blog. (2021, August 14). Evolve University. https://evolve-university.com/blog/the-ultimate-guide-to-muay-thai-knees/

Traditional Muay Thai fighting stances: the Art's bedrock. (n.d.). Muaythai. It. http://www.muaythai.it/traditional-muay-thai-fighting-stances-the-arts-bedrock/

WayOfTheArt (January 18th, 2023), Is Muay Thai Good for Self-Defense? (Street Fight). https://wayofmartialarts.com/is-muay-thai-good-for-self-defense/

Ways Of Martial Arts (January 24, 2023). Muay Thai Elbow Techniques And Combos https://wayofmartialarts.com/muay-thai-elbow-techniques-and-combos/

What is Muay Thai, Muay Thai History of training and fighting. (2008, December 30). Tiger Muay Thai & MMA Training Camp, Phuket, Thailand. https://www.tigermuaythai.com/about-muay-thai/history

Wilmot, A. (2013, July 2). Muay Thai. Awakening Fighters. https://awakeningfighters.com/awakepedia/muay-thai/

Wolcott, J. (2019, October 22). What makes Dutch kickboxing different from other striking arts? ONE Championship – The Home Of Martial Arts. https://www.onefc.com/lifestyle/what-makes-dutch-kickboxing-different-from-other-striking-arts/

Wolcott, J. (2021, July 10). Mastering the Muay Thai stance for beginners. ONE Championship – The Home Of Martial Arts. https://www.onefc.com/lifestyle/muay-thai-stance/

Yip, R. (2022, November 14). 3 common mistakes with your Fighting Stance. Infighting. https://www.infighting.ca/kickboxing/3-common-mistakes-with-your-fighting-stance/

Yokkao (2023), Essential Elbow Techniques In Muay Thai. https://asia.yokkao.com/blogs/news/essential-elbow-techniques-in-muay-thai

Yokkao (February 9th, 2021), How To Improve Muay Thai Skills https://asia.yokkao.com/blogs/news/how-to-improve-muay-thai-skills

www.ingramcontent.com/pod-product-compliance
Lightning Source LLC
Chambersburg PA
CBHW051850160426
43209CB00006B/1240